AN INTRODUCTION TO
THE PRACTICING HERBALIST

AN INTRODUCTION TO
The Practicing Herbalist

Meeting with Clients—
Reading the Body

SHARED BY
Margi Flint

AEON

First published in 2024 by
Aeon Books

Copyright © 2024 by Margi Flint

The right of Margi Flint to be identified as the author of this work has been asserted in accordance with §§ 77 and 78 of the Copyright Design and Patents Act 1988.

All rights reserved. No part of this publication may be reproduced, stored in a retrieval system, or transmitted, in any form or by any means, electronic, mechanical, photocopying, recording, or otherwise, without the prior written permission of the publisher.

Indication drawings by Matthew Wood or Margi Flint
Artwork by the author
Calligraphy by Kay Parent
Artwork photographed by Stacy Gormley and the late Jon Choate
Cover (Art Margi Flint, Calligraphy Kay Parent)

British Library Cataloguing in Publication Data

A C.I.P. for this book is available from the British Library

ISBN-13: 978-1-80-152-125-3

Typeset by Medlar Publishing Solutions Pvt Ltd, India

www.aeonbooks.co.uk

This book is an educational guide and reference and is not intended to replace the services of a physician. The author and publisher are not responsible for any adverse effects resulting from the application of information in this book. Either you or the professional who examines and treats you must take full responsibility for the uses made of this book. Before undertaking any self-care treatment, it is advisable to consult a licensed health care professional.

CONTENTS

FOREWORD   xiii
by Anne McIntyre

CHAPTER 1
About me   1

CHAPTER 2
Starting a practice   11
   Defining your philosophy   11
   Choosing your space   16
   Entering professional space   17
   Formula preparation area   18
   Creating an office space   21
   Organizing the desk area   25
   Using a computer   28
   Creating an herb closet   31
   The library   35
   The consultation room and classroom   36
   Laboratory: tincture preparation room   39

CHAPTER 3
Seeing clients	43
Compliance, identifying the constitutional body types	43
Vata	43
Pitta	44
Kapha	44

CHAPTER 4
Asking questions	45
The timeline	45
Sample of an intake form	46
Women	54
Men	61

CHAPTER 5
Understanding the endocrine cascade	65
Pineal gland	66
Hypothalamus: "the master gland"	72
Pituitary gland	78
Adrenal glands	81
Thyroid gland	86
Parathyroid gland	90
Hyperparathyroid (high)	92
Hypothyroid	93
Hyperthyroid	98
Pancreas	101
Ovaries	106
Testes	110

CHAPTER 6
Examining color	113
White	113
Green	114
Red	115
Gray	118
Yellow	118
Orange	119
Blue	119
Black	120
Purple	121

CHAPTER 7
Organ/body correspondences 123
   Stomach 123
   Small intestine 124
   Large intestine 125
   Liver 126
   Gallbladder 127
   Spleen/pancreas 128
   Lungs 130
   Kidneys 131
   Bladder 131
   Pelvic floor 132
   Heart 132

CHAPTER 8
Await indications of three 135

CHAPTER 9
Examining the face 137

CHAPTER 10
Examining the eyebrows 143

CHAPTER 11
Examining the eyes 145
   General eye condition 145
   Eye sockets 146

CHAPTER 12
Examining the sclera 151
   Color of sclera 151
   Pupils 152
   Client's view 152
   Below eyelid 153

CHAPTER 13
Examining the nose 157

CHAPTER 14
Examining the teeth, mouth, and lips — 159
    Specific indications of the teeth and gums — 159
    Examining the mouth — 160
    Lips — 161

CHAPTER 15
Examining the chin — 163

CHAPTER 16
Examining the tongue — 165
    LeSassier tongue diagram — 166
    The spirit of the tongue — 169
    Specific tongue indications — 171
    Coating on the tongue — 178
    Specific papillae indications — 179
    Thyroid tongue indications — 181

CHAPTER 17
Examining the fingernails — 183

CHAPTER 18
Examining the large intestine lines — 189

CHAPTER 19
Examining elimination — 193
    Stool analysis — 193

CHAPTER 20
Stool indicators — 199
    General — 199
    Color — 200

CHAPTER 21
Urine analysis — 203
    Urine color — 204
    Urine smell — 204
    Urine texture — 204

FOREWORD

by Anne McIntyre

It's hard to believe that it is nearly twenty years since Margi's first edition of *The Practicing Herbalist* was published by Margi herself. I remember that time well, and I recollect thinking at the time what a brilliant idea it was to give us the rare opportunity of a bird's eye view of a herbalist at work. I've always longed to know what other herbalists' practises are like, how they relate to the people who consult them, what their diagnostic tools are, what they put in their prescriptions and what their thinking was when formulating them.

It is fascinating how varied we all are as herbalists, each one of us creating an ever-evolving practice as we learn and develop from our life experiences: the people we meet, what we read and hear and the alchemy of this fusion in our ever-transforming hearts and minds. As Margi says, the unique gifts we have created from our own life experience are what we have to offer our patients.

I first met Margi in 1998 when I was invited by Rosemary Gladstar to speak at the International Herbal Symposium just outside Boston. That was the start of a new adventure in my life. I had never visited the USA before and my first encounter with this vast and varied country was with hundreds of herbalists! You can imagine what a rarefied view I must have had! They started the conference with an "opening circle" and with their warm sense of community and quite a different, somehow more earthy, way of being herbalists that contrasted with my hitherto rather confined experience of being a "clinical herbalist"; my eyes were opened wide, and I was hooked!

One of the first people to befriend me was Margi with her wonderful warmth and enthusiasm. She invited me to teach at Earthsong Herbals, her beautiful home and practice in Marblehead (which as Margi writes, is idyllic) and this was the beginning of a long friendship. We shared some wonderful times, and I loved going there sometimes twice a year to teach the students that she would gather, about the amazing world of Ayurveda. Margi, Rosemary and Deb Soule were instrumental in my being able to become part of the amazing community of American herbalists for over twenty years which I will never forget. I'm so indebted to Margi for the central part that she played.

Not only did Margi and I work and study together in those times, but we also had a lot of fun playing. I remember so well going out often to breakfast to a lovely café we would walk to. As we did, there were frequent calls of "Hi Margi". Everybody knew her, and you could see that they held her in high regard. She really was, and still is, the community herbalist and has been since the days when herbal medicine was considered much more eccentric and whacky than it is now. She was and is impressive! She has been the practitioner and the teacher for decades and yet she has always been the student too, not claiming to own her vast and profound knowledge and getting too attached to it, but acknowledging her debt to others in the field. I'm honoured to be among the teachers she acknowledges so generously.

Margi's descriptions of her practice are detailed and vivid, and even include which computers she uses and her invoice and banking systems …. all very helpful for anyone just starting out as they are setting up not just a herbal practice, but also a business that needs to support them if they are going to be able to practice their art sustainably. She accomplishes such a lot, seeing clients, making all her own medicines and prescriptions, teaching far and wide and I remember being impressed by how highly organised she was. Her home is lovely, the herb garden beautiful, and I remember fondly the distinct perfume of her dispensary!

The Practicing Herbalist covers so much ground and illuminates, in a way I find fascinating, Margi's unique way of practice for which she has gained well-deserved wide renown. She describes how she does a client intake and has included her case history form; I love her little helpful notes by questions on the form like "Varicose veins. Uterine Balancing Class (UBC), more bioflavonoids, Yarrow" and "Nose bleeds. Lack of bioflavonoids. Viral conditions. Nose picking, cut nails". She gives detailed explanations of the endocrine system, a unique description, to me, of how the varying colours of the body can be indicative of health imbalances, how symptoms in one part of the body can tell us about what's going on in another in her organ/body correspondences, and then she guides us through her unique way of reading the body. She begins this with the face and comprehensive diagnostic signs that I find very helpful and then page after page of tongue diagnosis—one of my favourite subjects! She continues with examining the fingernails, stool and urine analysis, pulse diagnosis and pulse testing and finishes with what she calls "quicksight confirmation"—a summing up in words and great illustrations of how to read the body—how the body in its great wisdom is telling us about other major body parts and their correspondences.

In *The Practicing Herbalist*, Margi has so generously opened her herbal practice for the world to see, and what a wonderful educational tool that is! Her chatty informal way of writing makes her descriptions of her world so easy to envisage, it is just like having a great conversation…though of course she is doing all the talking! Well, she is a wonderful and highly experienced teacher! And if, as she also says, our own personal experience with herbs and giving herbs to our clients is a far better teacher than anything we can read in books, this book is hugely valuable not only for new practitioners with not so much of their own practical experience, but also for others as they evolve their careers. The quest for insight and understanding about the workings of the human organism and its interrelationship with nature in all its magnificence is a subject as vast as the world that we will never finish exploring, which makes our profession just so much fun and perfect really! Thank you Margi!

CHAPTER 1

About me

I am writing this book for herbal practitioners. I constantly mention herbs and expect you to go to the many fine herbal books already published to research uses. I repeat myself in various sections of the book because that is the way I learned to hold on to information. You will read indications, hear stories, see tables, and view drawings. My intention is that the message sinks in on as many levels as possible. The herbs I mention along the way are suggestions, not absolutes. I certainly do not have all the answers. Herbs are to be tested and confirmed from your own repertoire and maybe mine. Jot down herbs you use successfully and draw lines you see on people into the pages of this book. Share new markings you discover with me! I hope you enjoy this book.

As practitioners, people will be drawn to us for the unique gifts we have created from our own life experiences. Sit quietly and view your life to see what your unique gifts are. What are your occupations, schooling, family life experiences, and personal experiences with health issues, therapy, life changes, and belief systems? What other experiences have made you who you are? Are you a serious person? Is laughter a big part of your expression? Singing? Physical therapy? Nursing? Mothering? Movement? Does science excite you? Value the work you have done and what you know. Do you just want the facts of the current complaint, or do you enjoy the life stories of clients? Is your gift sitting for twenty minutes and knowing the right herb? Are you a single-herb practitioner or a mixer? Be who you are, don't play a role. It is *you* that your clients are drawn to, so be yourself! Clients are drawn to you for your distinctive blend of knowledge and gifts. Let me introduce myself and tell you of my colorful background.

I am Margi Flint, and I have an herbal practice in idyllic Marblehead, Massachusetts on the East Coast of the United States. Marblehead is a beautiful seacoast town, that I have served, and it in turn has very nicely served me. I have a family practice. People of all ages come for consultation. All issues of health seeking and coping with disease, "being out of ease," enter through the doorway for herbal insights. That's where the term "Practicing Herbalist" came from. I practice as I learn each issue, each herb, each constitution, and each spiritual effect. I have had overlapping careers.

I have always loved to teach. I taught Head Start back in the sixties and early seventies in Roxbury and Jamaica Plain, Massachusetts. I loved those pre-school children and spent hours after work gathering supplies for them. I soon realized I was incapable of detachment. Teaching Head Start taught me to recognize the great potential in all people. It also opened my eyes to the great injustices in our world.

Teaching in middle school and high school taught me to learn not to peg people by appearance or by other teachers' opinions. Every human is capable of growth and the expression of joy. I began to feel the power of thought being the absolute greatest force we can call on.

I began my herbal path in the 1970s at the Gaia Herb Seminar, held at the 4-H Retreat Center in Ashland, MA. I was in art school, waitressing nights and weekends, and had left my Greek husband. Why did I leave him? Here is a good example of the power of thought.

I was unhappy. I felt trapped in a marriage. I was twenty-two. My sister Kitty's first baby, aged three and a half, had just died of cancer. I was looking for security in the bond of marriage. He was intriguing, from a foreign land and smooth, saying all the things I wanted to hear. None of it was true. After three months he said that we were married, I *had* to do what he said. Our differences grew, as did my feelings of fear and confinement. I developed symptoms. If I didn't leave the marriage my body would give me a route out.

A doctor sat across the wide expanse of his desk and papers and told me it was stress, some endocrine issue, or cancer of the pituitary.

I didn't even know what my pituitary was. He was cold. If it was cancer there would be nothing to do, a year and six months to live. I was to be X-rayed quarterly to observe changes in the calcium deposits around the pituitary and have mammograms to observe changes in my breasts. Well, as I sat alone in the back of a cab in rush-hour traffic along the Charles River I thought "I'm not staying with *this* man if I only have months to live!" I called my parents, packed up all my belongings and went home. I told no one of the diagnosis. I was the first in my family to be divorced. My parents helped me move and cooked my favorite meal.

I had undergone three of the four tests at Mass General Hospital. I had thrown myself into art school and was dancing every night to blow off steam. My symptoms began to disappear. I danced and drew. I was wild, and serious about my art. I was nicknamed "Mother Earth." I lived. I decided not to complete the tests. I felt I was impressionable. If they told me I would die then I would. So, I shifted into studying herbs, doing yoga, taking vitamins, seeing a chiropractor, an acupuncturist and reading spiritual books. I shifted away from alcohol and men in bars. I was actively raising my vibration. Meditation and the quest for a spiritual life began. I was creating myself with intention.

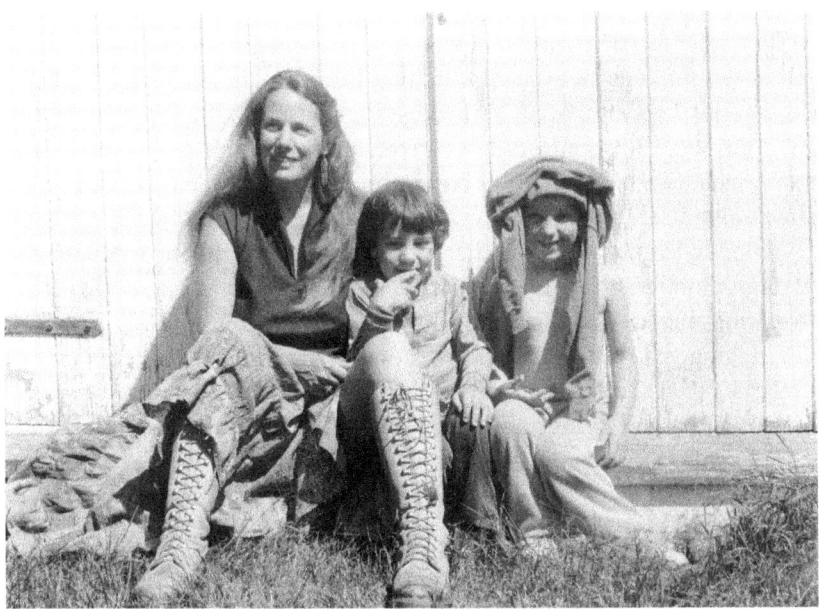

1986 Margi, Sarah, and Gabe

I taught art and Polarity Therapy in the seventies and eighties. I married again, a twinkly-eyed improvisational jazz pianist spiritual boy. Two beautiful babies were conceived and born at home through this union of the arts. We had a home full of music, creative juice, and the constant coming and going of friends. The guys would practice as I worked on etching plates and watched my Sarah, baby Gabe and little Hannah play or sleep. Hannah was James's only child, a five-year-old angelic being who fit right into our home life, tucked into bed with Sarah on those late nights of artistic fervor. Days spent pulling the little red wagon to the local beaches in between working. The marriage lasted all of five years, while those children I prayed for are souls with whom I continue to experience the depths of caring, sorrow, and joy. Their dad focused on his own path. What I asked for was children.

The Gaia Herb Symposium sounded interesting. There were forty-five or fifty people there, including the cooks and teachers, and we just thought it was huge. One teacher I met and fell in love with was California girl Rosemary Gladstar. We admired each other's lace petticoats. I showed her my portfolio of etchings. I soon began her correspondence course as a trade for my etchings. At the same time, I began my career as an artist.

At that same Gaia Herb Symposium, I met David Winston, a founder of Herbalist & Alchemist and the American Herbalists Guild. On the tables we sat, legs swinging, watching the people filter past us returning to their cars and lives after the symposium. As the last people left, we continued our comfortable conversation like kids back home on a stone wall. Since I had small children, and David lived in the garden state of New Jersey, I hired him to come to *my* house and teach me what I wanted to learn. I would gather a class together so that he would make enough money, and I would learn his wonderful blending of traditional medicine and science. He would also share one evening of talking about "Remaking yourself, the path to becoming human." The importance of dreams, stories, and personal ritual. Those evening stories were intimate kitchen and living room experiences that my kids still talk about.

Thanks to those two teachers and constant attendance at local seminars on herbal medicine, I began my path. Soon afterwards, I began attending all herbal symposiums within New England. Pam Montgomery held Green Nations Gathering in the Catskill Mountains. There, I discovered the diagnostic teachings of William LeSassier. I enjoyed many excellent teachers to excite my desire for deeper learning. Then herbs took over my life completely.

In 1989, the Women's Herbal Conference, brainchild of the late Gail Ulrich, was tiny. Those first years we camped on her rambling properties, holding classes under the shade of blossoming apple trees. We washed our dishes in rubber tubs and went without showers. The feeling was intimate and nourishing. My greatest gift to my daughter, Sarah, during her adolescent years was taking her with me. Sarah has joined me at the Women's Herbal since she was eight years old. I think the last Women's Herbal Conference had around 850 women participants. The impact of positive attitudes shared by these women has had a huge effect on the woman Sarah is today. The thoughts she carries in her heart toward moontime, budding, aging, and the variety of shapes in bodies has developed healthy self-esteem. She is all any mother could wish for.

Rosemary very conveniently moved East. I joined her first East Coast apprenticeship class. As a teacher, I look back on this inaugural class, composed of headstrong, opinionated women, and feel much sympathy for her. We were so anxious to share what we knew that poor Rosemary barely got a chance to teach. I can still see her in the front of the class with her patient smile, eyes raised to the ceiling, as one of us babbled on.

In my own classes, I sometimes get a chatty student who fills up a lot of class time. I remind them that they already know what they know…. Perhaps they might listen to receive the information they paid for. Closet by closet, floor by floor, hour by hour, my life began to be filled with herbs. The refrigerator had strangely packaged stuff in it. I remember Gabe eating a vaginal bolus thinking it was candy. Poor thing. The kids really were part of my learning adventures. They were the innocent recipients of my medicinal teas and early formulas. And they did survive.

I began teaching tiny classes: how to make salves, herbs for family care. Once I started teaching, I couldn't stop. I have a passion for herbs. I learned that I could enjoy my work and have passion for work that truly feeds my soul.

My now friend Rosemary Gladstar orchestrated The International Herb Symposium: Traditional & Modern Uses of Herbal Medicine. It was fondly referred to as "The World Church of the Holy Clovers." I was exposed to the top herbalists from around the planet. Awakening, inspiring and humbling.

I also labor-coached for twenty years. Being involved with birth, the first breath of life, has brought awe to my perception of life. I try to retain that wonder with each person I see. I am involved with people from before they are born, track them and enjoy their childhood and young man or womanhood. I have practiced long enough to see my baby clients enter their birthing years! I am a part of, not apart from this town.

My practice is very simple. I try to keep it pretty manageable. I tend to see one new client in the morning and one new client in the afternoon. Now that eight years have passed since the third edition of this book, things have changed. One client in the morning when I am fresh, and the duration of the day to accomplish the rest of life. Consults take an hour and a half, preparing formulas and billing another half-hour or two hours. Established clients guesstimate their revisit time in 15-minute increments. During revisits, we will alter their formula to adjust to the improvements or to switch the flavors or forms of treatment. The rest of the day I spend formulating, preparing salves or teas or tinctures for the office, preparing for classes, unloading herb orders, or answering never-ending phone calls and emails. The desk has an ever-growing pile of papers. Filing takes way too much time.

The practice helped to raise the kids too. I know that the energy of the herbs has permeated the entire house. The herbs have powers that are sometimes subtle and all-pervasive. The overall peaceful, yet at times hectic nature of the practice has exposed the children to aspects of human nature and imbalance they wouldn't see in a non-working home. They have been a part of my office often, either by running through it, or by helping to prepare products, their shining beautiful faces looking lovingly up at my clients. Ultimately, the kids would see what it's like to fall into ill health or dis-ease, and I think it has helped them to make better choices in their lives about what they will put into their bodies and just whom they want to hang around with. When they have pursued the temptations of their peers, they still have what they were raised on as a meter for their decisions. Don't get me wrong; we have not escaped the drama and heartbreak that all parents do. I did the best I was able to protect them, and I love those big babies no matter what frightening thing comes next. Life.

Polarity Therapy taught me the power of energy work to release the buildup of cellular memory in the physical body. I would recommend that anyone in the healing arts attune themselves to some form of energetic awareness. After a few years of psychosynthesis and studying Polarity Therapy, I married once more. This time I chose a man I thought was a good father, provider, and friend. Michael's daughter Emily joined our family on the weekends. Hannah needed a loving home, and I already loved her. My husband stated, "No, we don't have the money to feed another mouth." I said it was about a child, not money. Sometimes family is bound by more than blood. She moved in. Hannah grieved and completed high school and was loved by us. Some days, I cancelled everything and held her while she felt her emotions. Then we would walk or go out to the garden, and it would feel a little better each time.

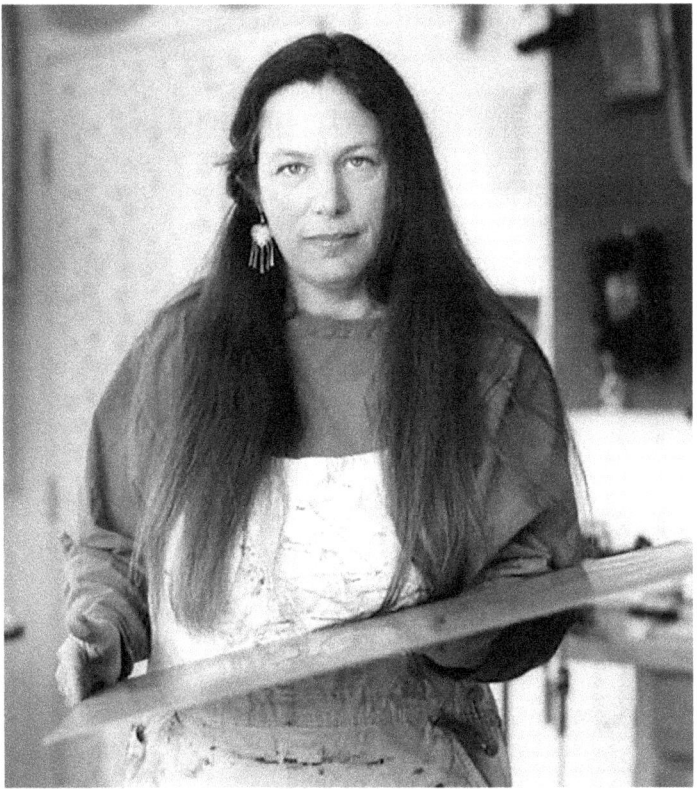

Margi's previous life as an artist

Etchings are created on wax-coated zinc plates, dipped in nitric acid, etched until the groove is the desired depth. The plate is then cleaned, inked, hand-wiped and run through an etching press to produce one print. The process is repeated until the artist is satisfied. My editions never exceeded 100 prints.

My career as a gallery artist was at a high point. The income from art sales carried my newfound addiction to studying and practicing with herbs, but my health was affected by the massive amounts of heavy metals in my system. That year my body created a kidney infection, the result of many toxins from making that beautiful artwork and some psychological toxins from another destined-to-failure marriage. Cobalt blue, cadmium, and zinc, not to mention benzene, asphaltum and a toxic array of solvents took their toll. Two months lying on my side, slowly, carefully breathing. Lots of intense pain with a side of broad-spectrum antibiotics. Not fun. And, the world went on without me. Those two months taught me to have compassion for people in pain. Pain is exhausting and takes the spirit to a low, and some days, hopeless, place. And so, at the peak of my gallery career, I walked away. My friends and family were aghast. Well, walk away I did. I stopped poisoning myself for "pretty." A few galleries continued to sell my work, which was a wonderful financial cushion. I learned that you can walk away from fame and fortune to follow your true path.

Creating the balance in health for people is as valid an art form for me as my etchings were. So, I really don't miss my art at all because I'm still doing it.

Thirty-three fascinating and revealing pages on this long life of mine continue in the full fourth edition of this book. I honor my teachers throughout these pages.

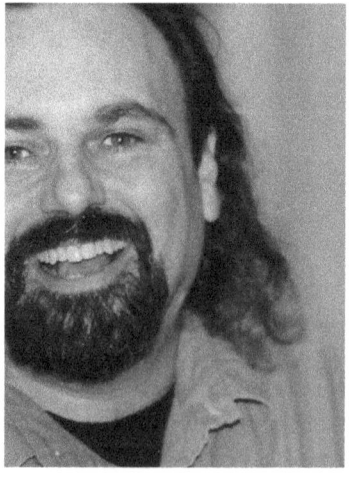

David Winston

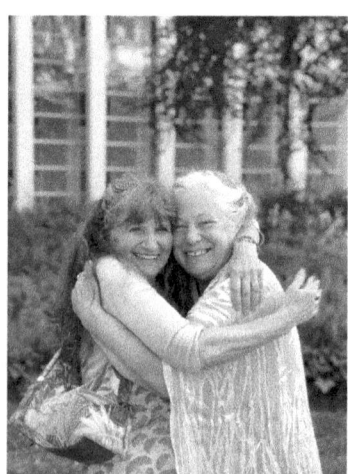

Rosemary Gladstar

ABOUT ME 9

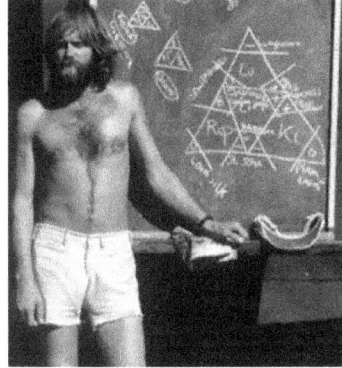
The late William LeSassier

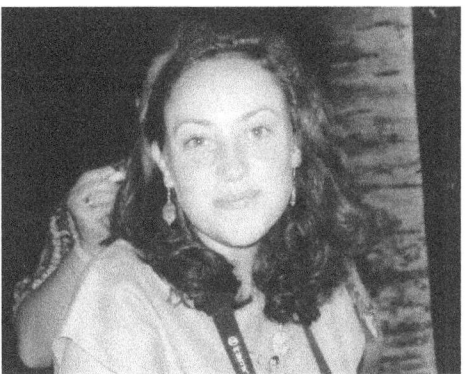
Daughter Sarah Matuza

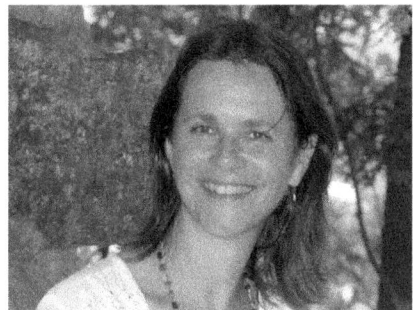
Annie McIntyre

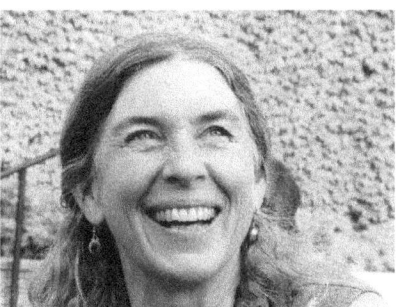
Kate Gilday

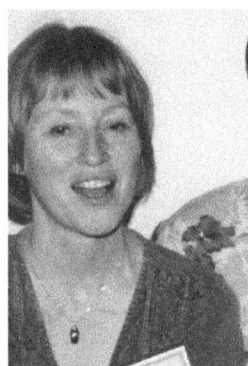
Phyllis D. Light

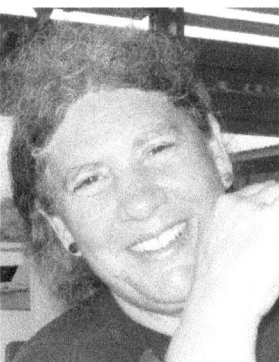
Karyn Sanders

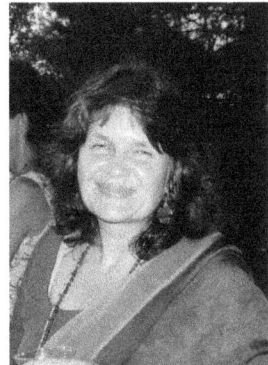
The late Cascade Anderson Geller

I attribute each teacher's information with a monogram. Please understand how difficult it is to remember who taught you what. We quote our teachers, who quote their teachers, who listened to the plants.

William LeSassier W.Le.	David Winston D.W.
Matthew Wood M.W.	Karyn Sanders K.S.
Phyllis D. Light P.D.L.	Annie McIntyre A.Mc.
Rosemary Gladstar R.G.	Cascade Anderson Geller C.A.G.
Kate Gilday K.G.	William Morris W.M.

All the plants (Invisible and felt deeply)

CHAPTER 2

Starting a practice

An herbalist knows when they are ready to start a practice, although sometimes the practice starts them. I have found several things that are helpful to have in place as you start your practice.

Defining your philosophy

A philosophy develops over the years. In retrospect I can pull some of these threads of thought together. I believe that when a client comes to me, they are ready to hear what I have to say. I shoot from the hip. I say exactly what is on my mind. I always try to express things in a kind way and am known for being blunt. We offer a sliding scale herbal clinic once a month or more, here at EarthSong Herbals, "Practitioners' Circle." Sliding scale means that the client decides how much to offer us for the consultation. They may give a few tens or hundreds of dollars. Practitioners recently sat with a talented woman with a darkly colored background. She had experienced ritual abuse throughout her childhood. She had successfully created multiple personalities and worked hard in therapy to untangle the emotions and memories. We discussed the various herbal approaches to her health issues. As the group lovingly focused on her every word she began to glow and shine the light of health. I asked this question "How does your illness serve you?"

I heard this question from Cascade Anderson Geller years ago on Sage Mountain in Rosemary Gladstar's Advanced Studies class. Cascade was teaching a class on How to do an Intake. I have found this one question to be most profound and most confronting. And sometimes people need to be confronted.

Back to my story. The lady cocked her head to the side, paused, and looked me in the eye. "This is the way I get loving attention." Yes, it is. To truly function in the world, each person must rely on his or her own spirit for love and healing. We practitioners hold some information, share some tips, and the healing is done by blending the herbs within the client. It is the client who takes the herbs in to heal him or herself.

The lady was afraid to be in relationships with people. Healers provided all the love and caring attention she craved, that we all crave. I encouraged her to jump off the precipice, create a loving relationship with her many inner selves, and join the world. Scary, yes, impossible, no. She called the next day to comment on my honesty and forthrightness. I appreciate that in others and am glad it is a part of me as a practitioner. She has taken her first steps into friendship with non-practitioners. People go forward when they hear their truth.

I believe that there is a cure in nature for all ailments. This beautiful planet has gorgeous plants all around us that have not even been exposed to the gray matter of our brains. The curative powers of the tiny Calendula flower are so abundant. "Liquid sunshine," as Matt Wood says, "for places where the sun don't shine," lymphatic drainer, skin healer and more. It seems that I learn a new use yearly. The quest for discovery is endless. Personal experience with herbs and herbs with your clients is a far better teacher than anything you will read in a book, including mine; they are the foundation of your practitioner knowledge. The puzzle of health imbalance is a challenge. And I do love a challenge!

There are websites to fill your head with the latest scientific research on herbs. It is a double-edged sword. Much of the research is done in a manner we herbalists would never employ. In vitro studies, the use of chemically standardized extracts, or use of isolated constituents are all, in my opinion, against Nature. These studies share with us the facts educating the medical minds. There is better research coming along. More input from herbal minds will in fact create better research. Know what is said so that you have an understanding of the comments your patients' doctors may make. If you read some of the studies you fill your brain with that information, as Bevin Clare said, and your mind will feel a little polluted.

I spent a day in the New Mexican desert with Doug Simons, who shared these words: "Know these plants as living people. We learned this medicine because the plants told us. We are like their children. Hear what they have to say, and our lives will change. Speak with a willingness to hear. Always honor the plants. We are here to become better relatives." Read *Braiding Sweetgrass* by Robin Wall Kimmerer. She teaches us that plants have named, talk about them as kin, or ki. Calendula, ki, is like liquid sunshine, kin can be dried in shade on screens with air circulating.

I also do honor the cycle of life. We, as herbalists, are able to make people more comfortable as they enter the next realm. The veils drop away. Death is natural. Sometimes it comes earlier than expected. Sometimes a person has done all the right things and they still become ill. This is the mystery.

Being busy, the phone ringing away, then times of quiet are also a natural cycle. Use those minutes when it is quiet to go within or out into nature.

I believe that the nutritional component to health is key. If our diet is fast food and soda the chance for maintaining good health is minimal. We can suggest dietary changes, gradually, allowing the client to adjust gracefully to new foods as they drop less desirable habits. I believe in all things in moderation, including moderation. We can suggest organic and locally grown foods, more food or less food. And then sometimes it is fine to enjoy a hot fudge sundae. Bless it and enjoy it. Presentation and education is everything. Our town had no organic food forty years ago. We have organics in every aisle of the local market now. The Farmer's Market is a huge event with music and demonstrations from restaurants as well as the vibrant produce from fifteen organically minded vendors. It is the main social event of the week. Supply and demand.

I believe that when a person is out of balance they manifest illness. First-hand knowledge. I can be incredibly dim when it is me that is sick. While writing the second edition of this book I had a visit to my doctor for a simple appointment. Right. She felt a lump in my breast, couldn't feel my ovary, and suggested tests. I resisted going (fear of radiation, fear of squishing fine lumpy, luscious breasts) and she expressed more, very sincere concern. Lots. So, for three weeks I was tortured by my own fears. This is pretty normal for health professionals who see lots of clients every day who share their horror stories about getting cancer. Yup: human, vulnerable, and scared. We have seen seemingly healthy people die right before our eyes. By the time I had the tests I had lots of other symptoms, all on the left side. After thousands of dollars spent (my new-fence money), I was declared healthy. As I was proofing this book, before my eyes, I read all of my symptoms. Diverticulosis. Who me? Clearly. Sometimes the person who projects calm and serene is pushing all of those tensions and fears inward. My own book! So, as practitioners we also become the client. And knowing that, realize that very intelligent people will come to you, and need you to explain every detail to them. We are all vulnerable and impressionable. They are with you for your help. Spell it out as clearly as possible. Now the book is in its fourth printing I know that all of the "I" issues are deficient intrinsic factor. Genetic as well as situational.

I believe we must teach environmental consciousness. We have been brought up on a false concept that you can "throw something away." There is no "away." What we buy in plastic, a can, or bottle that goes down the road in a garbage truck does not go away. Everything we do impacts on our neighbors. Products can either extend our lives or poison our planet. Imagine having to compost all that you purchase in your very own yard. This wonderful planet is small and living. We are a reflection of our planet. Take into your home, your body, only what you receive wholly. How does your body receive Styrofoam, plastic wrap, or color additives? How can you heal your uterus if you are consuming products that create birth defects in children?

If you want to have a voice about the direction herbalism is going you had better join in and vote. The American Herbalists Guild has been around since 1989. No complaining will be accepted from people who aren't expressing their opinions in a constructive manner. Stand up for what you believe in. Talk to the groups in your area when they gather. Whatever happened to political activism? It means filling out a ballot and mailing it in, or getting a like-minded soul to proxy-vote for you. If you vote, if you share your thoughts with your peers, change does happen.

Would you rather have a non-herbalist group decide your role as a practitioner? I think that herbalists tend to be solitary in their politics. That is fine; just try to creep out of your shell once a year. Richard Adams MNIMH in London, shared the definition of "compl e ment" with me. Complement is complete, "compl i ment" is a garnish. If I didn't understand the difference, I understand why many still interpret herbal practice as a garnish to modern medicine. I don't want to be a doctor, I am an herbalist, and proud of it. It really irks me when people refer to allopathy as traditional medicine. Traditional medicine *is* herbal medicine, the medicine of the Earth practiced in every country since the beginning of life on this wondrous planet. My training is unique in my field. Literally. Doctors' training is unique to medical institutions. Each has a very different model of training. We do not need to blend in; we can retain our individuality as a profession. With my Guild membership I am connected to other herbalists across the country. I go to the annual symposium, meet with other herbalists and share thoughts. If your organization does not change, or listen, and falls away even with your best efforts, well, start a new one.

And of course, continue educating yourself. Go to herb seminars, talks on plants, herb walks; learn about vitamins and amino acids and whatever else plumps up your knowledge base. Meditate with herbs. I have chosen to capitalize the names of herbs in this book as a way of honoring them as friends of mine. As my friend Russell Lane says, "Herbs are our friends."

When you're in the healing arts, any of the healing arts, you're giving away your heart all the time. So, as practitioners, I advise you, strongly, to set up a time where you replenish your heart, so that you don't give away your heart too much. Establish a time to sit and drink a cup of tea, write poetry, meditate, sing, jump up and down, walk in nature, sit in the dappled light of the apple tree, or whatever it is that brings you back to your center, back into your spiritual self, so that you don't give yourself away too much. I also believe that because we are exposed to so many horror stories from our clients' experiences that we become a little paranoid. If my vibration isn't high, I am more prone to worrying about every little ache or pain. As my therapist, the late Garbis Dimidjian said, "Worrying is like praying for what you don't want to happen." Find time to raise your vibration, relax your jaw, uncrease your forehead, drop your shoulders, and stretch those bones. Breathe. Isn't that what we tell everyone else to do?

The herbs have given themselves, their vital life force, for the continued life force on our planet. We receive nourishment from our Mother Earth. Return nourishment to Her. Compost. Take the strained herbs from your teas and poultices and return them to the Earth or you will not receive the medicine. Share this concept with clients. This thought is a First Nation belief that I have adopted, and I feel the power of its use daily.

So much of our societal life has separated us from nature. Isolation is a strong cause of disease. It is time to reintroduce the thought that we are all connected, each human, with each animal, with each plant, with each stone, bug, creepy-crawly, slimy, furry, hairy, fairy, with the air, water, fire, and the earth we walk on. Spirit is what connects us all. The silver thread, the web of life. Encourage clients to be in nature, to walk off the pavement onto the grass. To work out, and walk in, places that have clean air. Hmm, breathing deeply on the side of a busy road. I don't think that is healthy. To breathe deeply at the park or in the woods is a totally wonderful experience. Reconnect with nature.

I believe we are practicing herbalists. Our clients come to us and we practice on them. We learn by researching our herbs in books and more importantly in the field. We learn the relationship of plants to the people who take them in. We consider the energy of the plant and the energy of the person. All of that investment and devotion has a value. We honor ourselves on our journey by accepting an income that we are able to live comfortably on. We are all here to help each other live on this beautiful planet in a better way.

I believe there is always a way to help another soul. I don't believe in giving up. If I don't know the answer or haven't found success, I will refer my client out. I don't know everything.

What you believe today may not be your truth tomorrow. Information changes as the Earth changes in time. We as people change. Our perspective shifts. The plants change. And supplements, well, that information seems to change by the moment!

Choosing your space

I have a home office. It was important for me to be home with my kids. I wanted them to grow up with me. Is that a Freudian statement? They definitely got a dose of what Mommy does for a living. Sometimes they complained about all the people and all the students and having to clean all the time. Plus, they had to learn how to cook; a survival tactic for Mom-who-works-too-late. Now they have realized the benefit of having me at home for them and the gifts all those people gave to them and what good life skills they learned. Son Gabe and his wife Ali now own Avalon Gastro Pub in Kauai, Hawaii. To think he began on a stepladder pushed up to the stove cooking meals because I worked too late is a bit confronting. I would climb the stairs, see him look over his shoulder, spatula in hand smile and say, "Dinner's almost ready, Mum." Those early years of self-sufficiency paid off and transformed into a career for him.

In planning a home office, find someone who is very good at space planning; I suggest arranging a consultation. One hour with a professional may save you years of wasted time. For me, this person was Ted Sillars, my carpenter who created the office space. Ask around until you hear high recommendations for this skill. It took me years to figure out how to bring my office all on to one floor. I'm fortunate to have a house where I can have all my living area on the second and third floors and all my business on the first floor. This enables the rest of the household to carry on a quiet and unexposed-to-clients life. The first floor is all that has to be very clean all of the time.

Many practitioners have their office outside of the home. There are advantages to both situations. I will only share my experiences with a home office.

Entering professional space

When your clients first come into the office it's really nice if you have cleared the way for them. Have a neat entryway. As they come in, they will see that you are a normal, functioning human being, but you also have some order in your life. In that way, subconsciously, they'll feel as though you will have some order with them and be able to solve the riddle of their health issue. That sounds very logical. In real life the entry is sometimes full of boxes going out, the piles of boots and sandals, or winter coats on overflow.

I will walk you through my office. To the right of the entrance into the office, I have a large glass door. Now you would not know it was a door, because it is completely covered with little corkboard strips. Here I have flyers on the Women's Herbal Conference, Green Nations Gathering, the International Herb Symposium, American Herbalists Guild and other herbal gatherings, and flower essence classes with David Dalton. Also, there are flyers from practitioners in the area giving talks or seminars, herb-related or consciousness-related; community information on Yoga classes, dance, and meditation also goes onto this bulletin board. My clients love it. If I'm a little late it's no big deal. They can read and when they see something they are interested in we can just whip it right off on the copy machine, which is terrific.

This room is really the liver of the practice. Circulating through this room are the clients, herbs, products, money, bills, bottles, students, and transformation of all. It's important not to have a messy liver. This is where my assistant sits, when I have one, although she hardly ever gets a chance to sit. Most days I am my own assistant. I do pray for one devoted, gentle-spirited, efficient, compulsively organized part-time assistant.

In the middle of this room is a work island. This beautiful island conveniently organized with large drawers beneath the work surface. Structure. Beneath the drawers is my past life as an artist. The last of my etchings are in an architectural file cabinet, safely tucked away. Many of those etchings have been reproduced within these pages for your entertainment. Also in those files are the poster-sized facial diagnosis charts the late William LeSassier produced.

On each side of the island, I have four drawers. One drawer holds all my plastic massage oil bottles, with sprayers and flip tops. I am phasing out plastic and replacing with glass. The drawer beneath that has all the different sizes of salve containers: the metal tins and plastic flip tops, and the little, tiny lip salve jars. Then the top drawer to the right has all my wax paper bags to put teas in, masking tape to close them tight, and a roll of wax paper, large bags for putting orders together, large spoons and small, and a clean cloth, so that if there are any spills, I can whip it right out and clean up a mess right away. Beneath that I have my one-ounce, two-ounce, and four-ounce jars and a mixture of glass and food-grade plastic containers.

The opposite side of the island faces the shelves of tinctures. Each drawer is devoted to a different size amber or cobalt blue bottle with matching eyedropper, hard cap, or sprayer top. I have a case per drawer of half-ounce, one-ounce, two-ounce, and four- and eight-ounce jars. In the half-ounce drawer, I have a bag containing slim silver knives, forks and spoons, the tiny ones for pickles or lobster picks or baby utensils. These are for mixing essential oils into a client's products. Another has tiny glass vials for aromatherapy blends.

Formula preparation area

All my decorative labels are in a basket on top of the island. I love stickers. I love the reward system. The clients get to choose their own stickers for labeling at the end of their time talking. It is nice for people to get personally involved. It does kind of take you back to kindergarten,

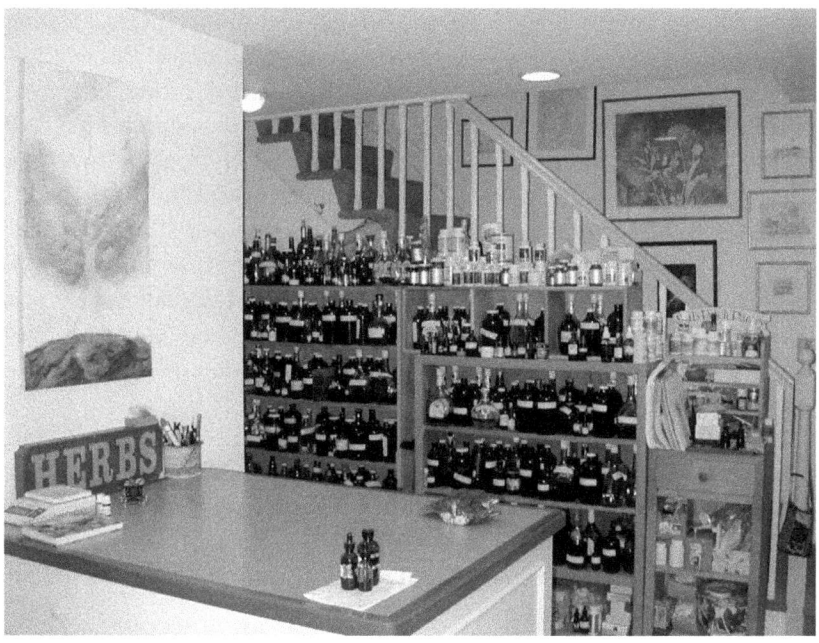

Formula preparation area

when you got a reward for being a good learner. Your clients are learning how to improve their health. Gold star! I have red, green, black, and blue permanent pens to write onto the labels. A mug in the basket holds markers. Always use permanent Sharpies. Other pens fade, like an old memory, soon to be a shadow of the past and useless on the shelf. Unmarked or faded labels on bottles are never to be used safely. The teas or capsules or herbs for long-term client use leave adorned with ingredients and daily dosage. I like to send a beautiful sticker home on its backing to be placed on the client's glass jar.

It is always interesting to see which image a person chooses. There are many books on symbols and their meanings to educate you. One particularly interesting book is *The Women's Dictionary of Symbols and Sacred Objects* by Barbara G. Walker. For instance, the image "butterfly" in Greek is Psyche, which means "soul" and also, "butterfly," the human soul incarnated as a butterfly while searching for a new incarnation. The Celts also believed in fly-souls and butterfly souls, which flew about seeking a new mother. In China, the jade butterfly is the essential emblem of love, a wedding of the souls. People are subconsciously drawn to what they are currently working on in their lives.

These images are received by the soul on many different levels. Healing is beautiful.

The island drawers are organized so that herbal products can go out the door easily. That way if I turn away from the island, I have all the tinctures I have prepared, alphabetically, on two three-by-four-foot shelves. On the top shelf I have all the "external use only" products.

Also, on the top shelf I have cordials and oversized storage bottles. So, I can grab a bottle of Dandelion Root tincture, turn around and pull out the right-sized tincture bottle for the client, fill it up, put a sticker on it, write the dosage, and put it on the end of the island. I then go over to my computer to write up the invoice. Organization makes the office run smoothly.

Above the tinctures is an air-filter/ionizer, which has run all day, every day, for the past forty years. Get a machine with a washable filter. Air quality is extremely important when mixing herbs. You inhale more pollen than most humans! You and your clients will breathe better. I have had clients with severe cat allergies sit peacefully for their consultation and not sneeze once.

The bottom shelf holds miscellaneous items, along with unopened bags of gelatin and veggie capsules for filling. Capsules and capsule makers are at the ready for apprentices. The torturous capsules. They can get right to work. A round hatbox contains all the prepared capsules that I have on hand. We have a lot of people with diverticulitis and colitis, and so I have to keep many prepared combinations on hand. Wild Yam, with Slippery Elm, Turmeric and Catnip caps. Slippery Elm to nourish, calm and heal, Turmeric for inflammation, antioxidant properties and to balance assimilation, and Catnip for the personality. Ah, what is a Catnip personality? Catnip people are the ones with a never-ending smile. When asked what is happening in their lives they smile and respond, "The house burned down, my husband just left and there is a little problem with my bowels." Catnip people wear a smile and stuff their frustrations and feelings inside. Give them Catnip and they return a week later with true reflections of their feelings. Chamomile people begin by sharing the long list of woes, whining all the way. "Give them Chamomile first to stop the whining, then they can come back," said the late William LeSassier.

Then I have more reference books, herbal and medical, and some prepared products for clients: facial toners and skin creams for young people and for us beautiful elder people. Ride and Glide and Radiant

Cream are probably the two most popular products to walk out this door. Radiant Cream is a wonderful product that has essential oils for rejuvenating as well as protecting the skin. It smells delicious. Ride and Glide is a "lower-lip balm" that originally was formulated for cervical dysplasia. It was just so wonderful that we decided to make it for everyone. Not to mention that our clients' partners are pleased to receive the benefit of the herbs! Compliance.

At the end of the tall shelves, I have a tall thin box with four cubbies. This holds larger supplement bottles, and new capsule makers for clients. When clients make their own capsules, they join in the process of healing. They also appreciate the time involved in making 200 caps. Atop this shelf sit business cards and too many tiny things that I never find a home for. This is just part of the clutter I constantly contend with.

All counter tops are cleaned with water and alcohol. I use a hydrosol of Rose or Orange and vodka. I use a clean white cloth. The cloth is laundered at the end of the day. No sponge shall ever touch my work or eating surfaces. Sponges are disgusting bacteria pits.

Creating an office space

Between the front door and desk there is a window. Outside the window facing the street is my carved wooden business sign "EarthSong Herbals." People can tell it's an office, so they walk in freely.

In front of the window are green wire florist shelves of all things that can go out the door in the hands of a client or student, used herb books, some products, and supplements.

Adjustable wooden shelves are between wire shelves and the entry. Prepared herbal oils: Comfrey, Plantain, Calendula, Arnica, Solomon's Seal, Wild Yam, Black Cohosh, Chaparral, St. John's Wort, and combinations frequently used. Beautiful oils that I use on a regular basis to make skin creams or salves and all the specific herbal products for clients. Kuumba cooks down exquisite coconut oil for your most extravagant gifts. These oils also turn over pretty quickly, but it's a lot easier if they are in alphabetical order on the shelf, ready to go. The lower shelf has green, white and pink clays, coarse and fine sea salts, Arrowroot, all the materials needed to make natural body care items. On that shelf I also have Black Cherry concentrate and Witch Hazel, all for preparation of products. Organize.

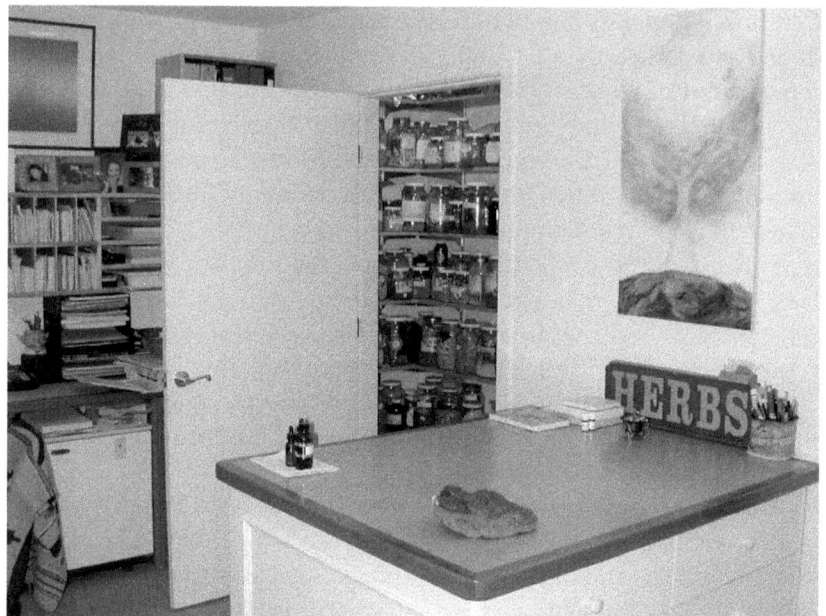

A view of the 4 x 12-foot Herb Closet

I have a small refrigerator beneath these shelves. This has really made the rest of my family happy. Refrigerators need to plug directly into the outlet, no extension cords. My family always found bizarre things in the refrigerator, so now all the bizarre things are downstairs. For instance, after spending a long night at a birth I might come home with a plastic bag holding the placenta. I place it in the freezer for safe keeping until the couple is ready to bury it with a nice tree planted over its high nutritiousness. Meanwhile, one of the kids could open the door to find a bag with a bright orange danger sign saying, "bio-hazard." What a world we live in. In the office refrigerator are the perishables, Evening Primrose oil, Coenzyme Q10, Vitamin E oil, all the probiotics, Royal Jelly, syrups, the hydrosols, and Grapefruit Seed extract. I have in there my Aloe Vera, cod liver oil and all the perishable essential oils like Orange Peel, Lemon, Rose, Jasmine, and Cypress. I keep a large stock of Rose Petal glycerite in there also. This little bit of magic adds a smooth loving taste and takes the edge off alcohol preparations.

On a top shelf I keep an embossed rectangular metal box with antiqued patina. Inside are blank intake forms and a large flat book, just the right size to write on. Tasha Tudor's *Book of Fairy Tales* serves as a

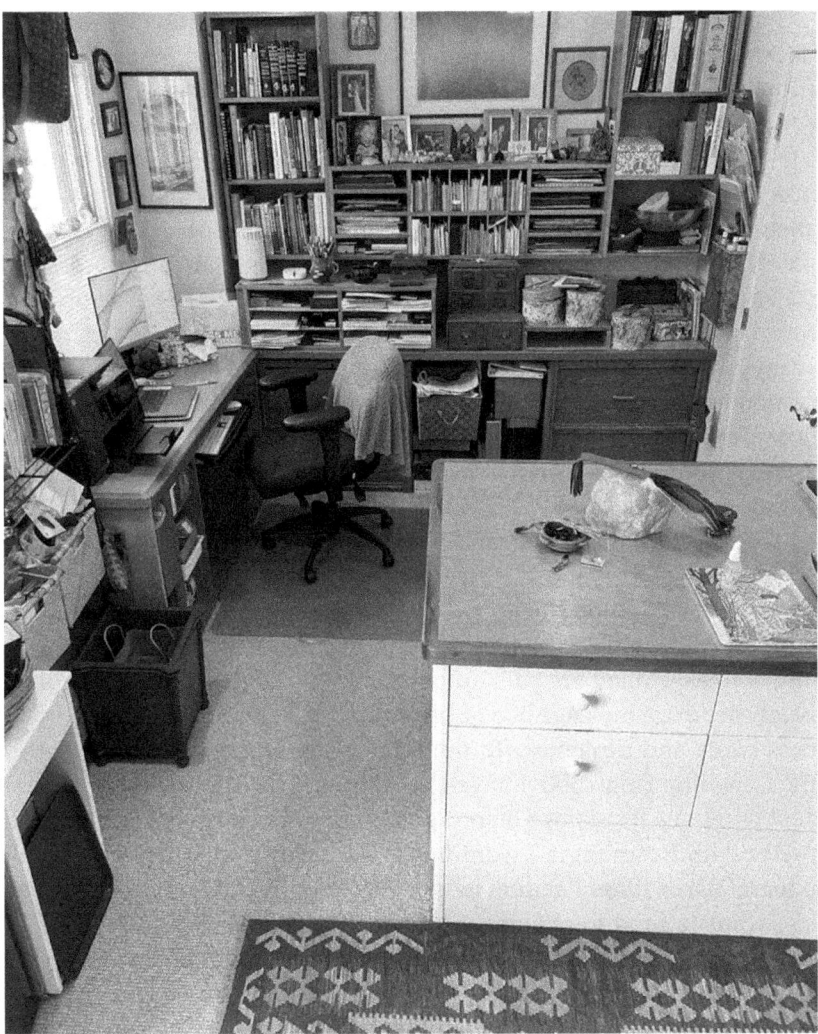

Desk area

lovely writing surface. I also have a few blank sheets of colorful paper to take my notes on. They are ready right at the top of that shelf, so that even if I'm really busy one day I can always just go to that shelf and grab one and not have to print another one out. My intake form changes as I do. If I don't print too many at a time my changes flow into the new form stored in the computer. I can see my clients coming up the stairs and entering the office.

I'm sitting here at my desk. The filing cabinets hold up the L-shaped desktop. The desktop is the same wood as the island, with the same trim as the nook. All unified. Easy to look at, less clutter for the mind. My MacBook Pro computer and an additional monitor sit on the desktop by the window. Heaven. I can actually use my desk for writing now that the hulk of the old screen is retired. To the left I have shallow shelves holding a few high-quality supplements. I use a Virtual Pharmacy, Fullscript, to suggest which supplements clients choose; they order their own and pay from home. I get a commission based on how much of a discount I offer. The phone has a speakerphone. Next to that is my precarious stack, the ever-growing pile of papers to read, correspondence, apprentice homework, some papers I think I must get to "one day." Don't ever put bills in this pile, they will not get paid. I have a Sonos sound system now, so music is there when I have the desire. Although, I must say, I work mostly in silence.

The beautiful mahogany and fir L-shape countertop was handmade. Mailing envelopes and cupboards are underneath the counter in an open vertical compartment. Behind the door are business envelopes with logo and envelopes that go with my checks, so that when I pay bills it's easy. Many are paid automatically through my bank. Simplify. Below are extra message books, bank receipt books, spare boxes of business cards and diplomas. To the right of the screen, I can see out to the flowering Dogwood. I have a two-drawer disc holder with vertical cubbies above for stamps on one side and bills to pay on the other. It is pretty with Roses on it. I want to have a positive association with bill paying. All of those vendors help me to have a more efficient practice, so I want to send the payment off with Roses. I have become fond of order-through pretty containers. If I don't put my bills in the pocket they disappear among the fluttering papers.

A folder file in the corner perches atop a wooden U-shaped shelf that was handmade for me. Colored file folders hold the current year's classes and seminars where I will be lecturing and my list of good and bad doctors. That's right. I keep a list of doctors, body workers, and therapists that people love and those with whom people have had bad experiences. I have a file of research papers I have good intentions to read, and a folder for CEUs for the Guild. Under the folder file are my checks to feed into the computer. To the side against the corner wall leans my notebook to log computer registrations, virus data, and questions for my techies. Yoda holds my calligraphy and other favored pens.

I have a rotating holder for pen, paperclip, marker, highlighter, and pushpin holder. The phone message book holds 400 duplicates. I can staple the dated copy into a client's file when they call with updates concerning their health.

Organizing the desk area

Rounding the corner on surface of the counter is a HP printer, scanner. Very nice. Like printing with champagne, though. It perches on a wooden upside-down U-shelf. Under that I have my bank stamp for deposits, scotch tape, and a stapler. Beneath it Mom's old-fashioned adding machine that prints the figures on paper tape. The old and the new. Lovely wooden cubbies hold colored and decorative letter-sized paper and checks for the computer. Beautiful "train cases" hold essential oils, or class materials for my latest favorite class to take on the road. One box has aphrodisiacs, chocolate soap, essential oils to relax and stimulate, a Sandalwood fan, and outer and inner massage oil. There are four to five of these boxes lining the wall. I have a large set of nested stainless mixing bowls. Then a stack of papers waiting to be filed. Waiting and waiting. Lastly, next to the wall of the herb closet are my personal essential oils kits. They reside in beautiful flowered train cases. So sweet, so small, so just-another-box, full of hundreds of dollars' worth of five ml bottles with "pitons." A piton is the plastic orifice cover that allows only one drop at a time to leave. Highest-quality essential oils need to be protected from the elements and the vibrations and infrared rays of people. I love Aromatherapy. Over the years I have developed a more sophisticated nose thanks to my teachers Mindy Green, Linda Patterson, Kathi Keville, and David Crow. The curse is that I now pay more and tolerate no oils that are chemically distilled.

Beneath the counter is a double file cabinet that holds all my tax-related business receipts. This includes the bills from utilities, phones, office expenses, mortgage, insurance companies, shipping and handling, various banks, credit card receipts, medical expenses to deduct for the year, donations, sales, state, property, excise, and federal tax papers, and cash receipts. I keep a file for my federal ID number. In that file are my Massachusetts resale forms to be sent out to vendors who otherwise would charge me sales tax. No sense in paying it twice. That too is alphabetical. Keep all receipts. If you keep track of all your business doings, the Internal Revenue Service will not be a worry. It takes twice as much energy to lie. Be in a place of integrity.

In the right-hand file cabinet, I had a whole section of handouts for clients. (I now print these off from the desktop folder, "Handouts.") I have handouts for people who have high cholesterol, diets for stones, inspirational articles, lots of herbal protocol directions, such as how to make an herbal oil, tincture or tea, information on dairy, ear, nose and throat issues for children, educational information on Chaga, Reiki, or the urinary system. Relationship communication skills, meditation practices, sacred rituals, and recipes. Folders for these handouts are in that file so that at the end of the consultation I don't have to repeat all this information to a person. I can just hand them this flyer, this little handout, and they can go home and read it in peace. Oftentimes they've received so much information in an hour and a half's consultation that they would be a little on overload if you added more. This way it's written down and they can look at their diet for high cholesterol, and stick it up on the refrigerator, or whatever, and it allows their brain to relax a little bit.

I have all my blank file folders for clients and teaching. I like colored folders. They make me happier than manila. I use a surge protector to plug all the computer plugs into. Now I have a battery backup NAS system just in case the Cloud blows away or my computer crashes. All the books unpublished are worthy of saving. We Flints have this attraction to lightning. I like to shut it all down when the thunder rolls by.

Underneath the far shelves is a section in the file cabinet for business-related information. I have one whole section on classes that I teach, either lectures for traveling to hospitals and seminars, or classes for my apprentice programs. I continue to update these, but it's nice to have a hard copy to look over before you go back into the computer and change the class as it evolves. I have warranties on the various machines I have bought for the office. I have a file of sappy letters from family and friends (client letters I keep in their file in the library), funny email jokes for future classes, class records, quizzes, and syllabi for the college courses I teach. Important papers. In this fourth edition of life I have ended teaching apprentice programs, running clinics and long weekly courses at colleges, so all those files are free to be filled with more personal papers.

I had upper shelves built above the desk on the widest wall. They are fantastic. They have cubbies for cards and envelopes, lots of cubbies, twelve little cubbies, and in there are brochures on where to buy products, like Mushroom Harvest. I save all of the other teachers' flyers on classes, and if people say, "I'd like to study, where else could I study?" I can say, "Oh you can go study with Emily at Sage Mountain, or go to Nicole Telkes at Wildflower School of Botanical Medicine in Texas, or Deb Soule's Avena Institute, or to New Hampshire to Misty Meadows with the joyous Wendy Snow Fogg." Watch the birds in the fields while you learn! I love my students and also believe in studying with more than one teacher. I have everyone's flyers up there, and correspondence course information. That way I can pass on information to all that enter.

I have lots of different types of gift cards, a whole section of herbal photographs, and then I have eight cubbyholes that go the long way. Those flat slots are filled with all my copy paper, all the colored paper, and my business stationery—all the beautiful paper; easily accessed to make copies or use in my printer. In that way I can see immediately what I want and where it is. Then I have another huge stack of things I'm supposed to be reading, which I seem to never get to.

To either side atop that I have two large bookcases, which go nearly up to the ceiling. They hold some reference books. I have a medical dictionary: Thomas Bartram's *Encyclopedia of Herbal Medicine*, then Thomas Easley and Steven Horne's *Modern Herbal Dispensatory*, Matt Wood's *The Practice of Traditional Western Herbalism*—his books must be close to me—and now Christa Sinadinos's *The Essential Guide to Western Botanical Medicine*. Weight-bearing exercise. Of course, Rosemary Gladstar's *Herbal Healing for Women* and all others. Amanda McQuade Crawford's *Herbal Remedies for Women* and *The Herbal Menopause Book*. Her recipes are so good the book is falling apart. Sajah Popham's *Evolutionary Herbalism*. Also on this shelf are books that I commonly look through for making products, like Dina Falcone's *Earthly Bodies & Heavenly Hair*. Then a whole bunch of books on diagnosis of tongues, fingernails, face—really any book that helps fill in the gaps in the mystery. Llaila O. Afrika's *Complete Textbook of Holistic Self Diagnosis* is the first I have read addressing dark-skinned humans. It is one of the most comprehensive diagnostic texts I have ever seen. Even though I am light-skinned, his gathering of wisdom is pertinent to all. What a surprise. We are all connected.

I have herbal information and supplement information, for easy reference. There is an entire shelf of skinny notebooks that hold teaching notes for the various classes I lecture on: Reading the Body, Hospice

Care, the Endocrine System, Ambiance and Sensuality, Living with Cancer, Clinical Practice Pearls, Affirmations for Herbal Choices. Each year the classes shift, the notes change; the wisdom is reworded between archival plastic pages. I have IN/OUT trays holding notes for the books and projects I am currently working on. Last, but not least, I have my formula book. Lots of precious cargo on those gorgeous wooden shelves.

Photographs of my teachers flow across the mid-section: my parents, my kids, Rosemary, Ian White, and of course William LeSassier, dear Tim Whiting, goddesses of various traditions, herbs from ceremonies past, and a few bears, elephants, and dragonflies.

The ceiling has six brass and glass shades with full spectrum lights that shine down on us all day or night. A little bit of that purple hue makes a huge difference in mood and the appearance of everyone's complexion. Living here in the Northeast makes for a lot of gray days. Full spectrum lights increase happiness and decrease depression. I spend many hours in these rooms and want to treat myself the best I possibly can.

Using a computer

I own two computers, both Apples! I started with a Desktop and worked my way up to a bigger one. Too big. The screen was for gaming and gave me a stiff neck. That went to my daughter Sarah, a teacher, during The Great Isolation of 2020, now 2023. Actually, she has the last two desktop versions because the kids needed virtual classrooms as well. Currently the MacBook Pro is permanently connected in the office and the Air travels with me. QuickBooks Pro Online is my accounting program. QuickBooks has a decent system made for small businesses. Your chances of infection from viral or worm infections are much lower on Macs. Plus, you can purchase Apple-friendly power point presentations from Lisa Ganora on the Phytochemistry of Herbs. Buy your computer from a reputable store that includes lessons, and a fabulous warranty. I have a number of IT geeks who I adore, who care for the well-being of my office. To detach my computer and drive it away to be among the missing for days on end doesn't work unless I am also away from my work.

The computer mantra is "Back up. Back up. Back up." Buy an external hard drive, back up to the ethers, and have an automatic backup. Back up every day. But do, oh do, back up.

I'll go over to the computer and fill out the invoice for my client. QuickBooks has invoices and cash sale units, and it does inventory and all sorts of things, which make your life very easy. Easy if you fill the information in properly. For example, I can just type in "one ounce Dandelion," and will see a list: Dandelion leaf, Dandelion root, Dandelion tincture, and Dandelion flower oil. This makes it easy for me to just use the little arrow to find the right one and then the price I've already fed in. As soon as I make or buy a product, I figure the price by ounce and enter it, so that an ounce price comes up first. Then all I need do is put in the quantity, and the program calculates the price for that amount. I don't have to decide what the price is in front of the client. As you order herbs and products, input the prices, a little at a time. In my early years, clients would come, and of course I would fall in love with all of them by the end of the hour and a half. I wanted to give them everything, and I did. I think that I probably lost thousands and thousands of dollars a year, because it was hard for me to determine a price in front of someone, and I hadn't taken the time to figure out my overhead into herb sales.

When you make a product, you really do need to weigh out how many ounces of menstruum and herb you use, how much time it took you to make that product and what the cost of the bottle and the label is. If you buy alcohol, that is an "expense" under the "income" made from herbs. In this way you get an idea of how much profit you may be taking in. And you need to figure it all into your pricing, including, if you are renting, your rental price. You add up all the square feet of the home and divide by the portion used strictly for business. In my case I deduct a third of my mortgage and utility costs for the business. Wouldn't it be nice to also deduct the kitchen? Yes, but I use that for home use so I can't. So, there's a certain percentage of each day's income needed just to *meet* your living expenses, which is a rude reality. It's expensive to run an office.

An "invoice" is given when the client doesn't have a check or cash with them—they take the bill and mail you a payment. A "cash sale" is when they hand you the payment in cash or check. If you take credit cards it is easier for people to come up with payments. The rates vary, but it is usually between 3½ percent and 5½ percent of the total sale. The bank will offer various plans. This is a good idea if you have lots of people who charge. Currently I send the invoice out through QuickBooks, the client pays from home, then I ship their herbs. Safer. If you think of these banking expenses as the cost of doing business, you will sleep better.

Collecting money is done from the "overdue invoices" list. Scary. When people have forgotten their checkbook or are short on cash, they get an invoice and are expected to send the money in to the office. Sometimes I don't get paid. That's called a "bad debt," and it is. It is bad karma to not pay any caregiver. I figure that after a few letters and a phone call I will take the deduction at the end of the year for my taxes, and they their karmic deduction. So be it. Right?! No more. Come to clinic if money is an issue, all bills are paid before I hand the herbs out now. I want time to play, not chase down payments.

In the past my students made payments over the duration of their class times. I prepared an invoice with the total amount of the program and go to the "receive payments" section of the software program when they made installments. It always looked as though thousands of dollars were owed to me. Sometimes they were. Some days the mail came, and hundreds of dollars magically poured into the office. Great. Some days I forgot that the Universe is full of abundance, and I sat at the desk and cried. When people don't honor their agreements, it hurts. It's human nature.

On the invoice I include the herbs and portions by ounce. I wish I had grown up in the decimal system, so round. When the client has the proportions, they are able to create their formulas wherever they go. Be sure to write down all of your suggestions on separate papers. Two copies. Notes for Clients include their name, date, and all instructions on foods, movement, herbal instructions, and affirmations. Infused, decocted, the number of drops in water, under the tongue, or into a water bottle, teas or salts into baths, poultices, steams or whatever your protocol requires. You know all the information; it is all new to them. It is very hard for them to retain all the information once they walk out your front door. Any additional handouts are handed over with the bill. A permanent record. Keep a copy of the invoice in their file. Believe me, you will refer to these frequently. Keep good records!

I put all of my business expenses on to my credit card. This gives me mileage on the airlines, so that when I have a business trip or I want to take the kids on a vacation, I can use those miles. Hard-earned fluff. This also logs your business expenses much more accurately. The online version makes it simple for my accountant to merge statements into my account. No more endless hours copying line by line from all statements! Freedom! Be sure to take advantage of the program.

One icon list holds all "vendors" that I purchase products from; all phone numbers, addresses, and employee contact names for herb companies, supplement companies, and book dealers are at my fingertips. I buy glass and plastic bottles, hundreds of dollars of bottles a year from Burch Bottle, SKS or Andler Bottle. Shipping invoice paper I file in the company folder, and in that way I have a double record of everything I've bought. If I need to look back to it or show apprentices how much they can save by chipping in on a case, I can easily reference that. I have a computer record and a paper record. This is probably untrue now. Most cards are online so my forest waste is less.

Why did I keep all that paper in file folders? This is a flashback to when I had an HP computer …. Because one day you may forget to back up. And a computer virus or worm will enter into your little box, and away will go all of your carefully loaded files, invoices, records of all kinds. Yup, a nightmare. If you have an Internet connection, you are vulnerable. Worms and virus invasion from unknown outside forces. Files corrupted. Horrible language, eh? Herbs won't help. A firewall will. Maybe. The creepy worms got in from attachments, were quarantined and slowly eliminated six months of my bookkeeping. Twice. That cost me thousands in time, lost unpaid invoices, redoing monthly accounting and outside computer help. Time Machine backup to the Cloud, some to Dropbox and everything to the battery Naz backup. Go ahead, call me paranoid.

So, even though it goes against my nature I have become vigilant with email connection. I don't open attachments until I know the person is virus-free. I don't open emails that give my stomach a twinge. I check return addresses for scams and cons, and still fall prey when too busy. I unplug the cable and call for my computer-genius as soon as I notice the computer is slow or odd in any way. I consider it cheap insurance against the insane ones of the world.

Creating an herb closet

It was well worth the money that it took to invest in having a nice herb closet made. The first herb closet was our kitchen pantry. The new space is twice as big. Mine is four feet by twelve feet. Heaven. It's quite beautiful. Clients love to come in and just stick their head into the herb closet and smell the beauty of all those herbs. They feel rejuvenated and healed by just being in the presence of herbs. They feel the magic.

During construction of the herb closet I had a shelf built into the new wall that leads to the library. Closet walls are six inches deep and do not need to be sound-proof; wasted space. Ted Sillars did the design and construction. He has a mellow nature and his vibration is part of his work. Ted built in between the studs a gorgeous hardwood nook with adjustable shelves to hold essential oils, skin creams, massage oils, plus Lice Away (essential oils to be added to shampoos for all the local schools that get lice outbreaks), and other small items we make for clients. Everything ties together, very aesthetically pleasing. It's a terrific use of space. If you are going to do any construction, think about shelves you can build in between the studs for these small herbal products. Ted also designed the island, counters and upper shelves, built-in library shelves and my deck. I am glad his vibration is here.

The closet is large enough to hold all of the glass jars for all of the herbs, plus a top shelf for an extra pound of almost everything. The turnover is so quick in the office, and I need to have the herbs on hand, readily. Sometimes I just don't have time to wait a week or two for an order to come through. Individual herbs in gallon jars take the bulk of the space in the herb closet. I try to only keep gallon jars and half-gallon squares. They are wonderful, because the squares can stack on top of each other, and that way herbs that are very expensive, bought in smaller quantities like Chinese Red Ginseng, are less exposed to oxygen. A small quantity of herb in a large jar is too much oxygen exposure. Ages too fast.

If women are on their moontime, I ask that they not enter the herb closet. All the other days, women can cook and clean, make medicine, and make love. These are beliefs I have adopted from David Winston— some of his First Nation trainings resonate with me. The power of a woman shedding her uterine lining is great. She releases all of the energies and issues of the month that need to be released, for herself and for her partner. She is *so* powerful at bleeding time that she might pull away the healing energy of the herbs. Moontime is time for rest, introspection, and paperwork, a time to honor yourself for all you do by resting and receiving.

One end of the herb closet is devoted to prepared teas and herbal supplies. I have prepared base formulas, and then for each individual client I can add the specific herbs to the foundation of this formula. Quite an effective way to cut down on wasted time in the office. I have lots of formulas: one for the urinary tract, one for heart support, and one

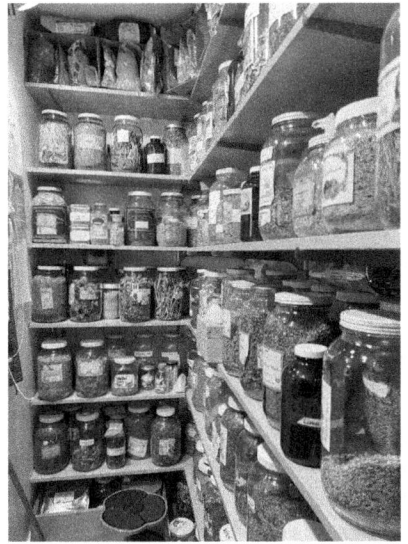 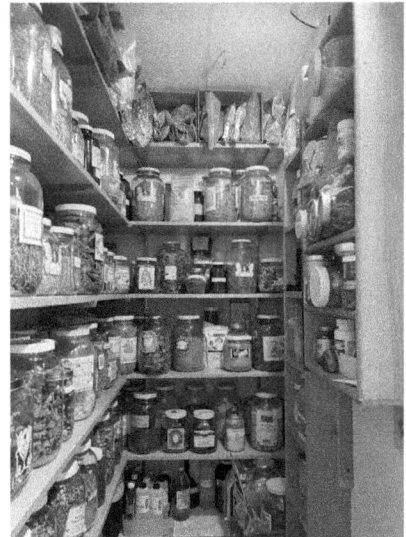

Herbs to the left   Herbs to the right

The Herb Closet

for colicky babies or upset stomachs (it's basically Rosemary Gladstar's after-dinner tea, a nice digestive aid and calming tea). It's nice to have that convenience.

My first herb closet was our pantry. The food was distributed elsewhere. I had roots on the bottom shelves, leaves and flowers in the middle, and barks and seeds on the top. When I began teaching, I realized that students didn't know which was a flower, root, or bark. The closet quickly became a mess. So, I succumbed to the alphabet. I still have to sing it. I will say that the alphabet is a great way to organize; I resisted it for years, having that rebellious spirit. Then you need to decide if you will go by Latin or common name. Ah, decisions, decisions.

One section is filled with Ryan Drum's wondrous Waldron Island seaweeds. Ryan is the best wildcrafter in the USA. No prejudice at all. He has trained others to also wildcraft consciously. The vibrant life force of wildcrafted herbs from Ryan, Matthias and Andrea Reisen of Healing Spirits, Kate Gilday and Don Babineau of Woodland Essence, Nancy and Gracie Phillips of Heartsong Farm, and Mel and Jeff of Zack Woods Herb Farm are beyond compare. Mountain Rose Herbs and Frontier, Starwest Botanicals, Frontier Cooperative, and Etsy fill in constantly. I love to bring two jars of an herb, let's say Hawthorn leaf and flower, to a class. Those that were lovingly prayed for, thanked, harvested at the correct time of day, correct weather conditions, in the correct growing season and dried with knowledge—well, they shout out their essence. The vibration is intact. They last longer in your closet. They work better in your formulations. They hold the powerful nutrients, and their energy is ready for us to receive. In the other jars I will show commercially grown, shredded to an unrecognizable sifting of packed herbs, lifeless in comparison. Learn to recognize quality.

On the very bottom, the floor, I have extra gallons of Apricot, Coconut, and Jojoba oil. I have pounds of Shea butter that is so buttery and euphoric. I like to get Shea butter from this great gal Margi in Texas. Organic Cocoa butter, and Coconut oil are just waiting for preparation of essential oil products, or cosmetic products. Beeswax is always on hand. Beeswax comes from Andrea and Matthias Reisen at Healing Spirits, gorgeously dark aromatic Beeswax in blobby chunks. The more Propolis that finds its way into the wax the better. Immune help through cream. Yummy.

I have a little wire rack that rolls and has the extraneous stuff that I, for some bizarre reason, cannot fit on any of these shelves (which were built to hold way more than I could have imagined at the time). So, make your closet a little bigger than you think you need. Okay, a lot bigger. I do think that the herbs need to be behind a door, so that they can have their own energy and be apart from the energy of the comings and goings in the office. In this way they retain their own personalities, plus they are, of course, away from light and heat. The herb closet does create its own temperature, and I do have crystals in it, and I do pray in there to try to maintain the high energy of the room.

Another choice would be to send your clients to a quality natural foods store for their herbs. This will save you investing thousands of dollars in jars, herbs, and oils. Plus, you can avoid the horror of miller moth invasion. Those little gray moths can devastate your highest-quality herbs in no time.

The herb closet door has a little button in the hinges. When the door is shut the lights automatically go off! Wonderful. No more cooked herbs overnight. Just inside the door on the wall is a clipboard for noting herbs, essential oils, carrier oils, and other inventory to reorder. Tinctures needing to be made are constantly noted and scratched off. I also have a weights and measures chart beneath the list. I just never retained those ounce-to-gram–to-liter numbers in my head. I hold a lot of information up there and sometimes you must accept memory nudges. On the wall is a photo of the late and spectacular Tim Whiting smiling behind a massive Poke root. It is my closet and full of love.

The library

Client files are in a vertical four-drawer file cabinet in this back room. Each drawer has a label, A through E and so on, to divide the masses. The folder tab has the client's last name first and first name after a comma. Colored folders help me find client names more easily. Place the start-date on the outside of the file. Client files where seven years have passed without rebooking are shredded. I have a digital camera now. I began photographing clients and keeping their face right inside the folder so that when they call or have an appointment, I have one more way of remembering who they are. It is also a way to document major changes in the face, tongue, or nails with an additional photo. I used to remember everyone, and their entire medical history. Now, hundreds of clients later I need a memory jog and review of their folder. Four drawers full of clients makes for a lot to remember. Now when I see a health practitioner I don't expect them to remember every detail of my life. I come prepared to remind them of the important details.

Entering the library, on the right are skinny shelves, one jar width, with small bottles, jars, shakers, and more.

The "coat closet" holds cases of extra jars, bottles, caps, lids, and powder containers. Stacks of plastic crates within hold packing materials, shipping boxes, and tissue paper.

I removed the doors leading out, and had the back porch winterized. This left the central bearing wall intact, allowing for waist-to-ceiling bookshelves. Back-to-back is a set of wooden bookcases, which extends the wall, adding an element of privacy from the neighbors. The library side holding a media center with audio or videotapes for apprentice or client rental. The TV, DVD, and tape players are upstairs, well used.

Ted Sillars returned and created built-in gorgeous shelves echoing the heart them from the deck he designed right outside the back door. I tend to organize by grouping, not author: women's health, children's health, pregnancy, all that sort of thing. General health books from the great masters: Bernard Jensen, Culpepper, King, and Dr. Christopher, as well as from our modern masters: Rosemary Gladstar, Christopher

Hobbs, David Hoffman, Annie McIntyre, Michael Moore, Michael and Leslie Tierra, Sajah Popham, and Matthew Wood. Oh, the list goes on and on. Forgive me for not listing each author. I try to collect books written by herbalists, not patchwork writers of other people's information. There are sections on essential oils, flower essences, materia medica; some books on pressure points, meridians, other healing modalities. I feel like a bookstore sometimes. And I always want more.

The family's eighteenth-century "camp bed," a rope-bed with the longest screws ever and a canopy graces the center of the room. This was my great, great, maybe another great grandfather's bed when he was the aide-de-camp to President Zachary Taylor. They would take it apart, place in a wagon and move on to the next battle. My Mom was gifted it, and she and my Dad never had a battle under those sheets. Now it is my guest's or mine on hot summer nights. I hope to absorb all the knowledge from the books while I sleep. The shelves closest to the light and pillows are all on aphrodisiacs and love play. Above them Native Knowledge, beside those esoterica on colors, energy work, astrology, delightful herb-related novels, and palm reading. Much better than a magazine.

The old porch became my hide-away writing area. North-lit yet sun-filled windows all the way to the corner, a glass door, and another window. In my grandmother's writing desk are projects I am currently working on, art supplies nearby. There is a peachy velvety armchair gifted from Ryan Nolan in the quiet corner to snuggle in and enjoy blissful reading or peaceful Zoom classes. I look out to my gardens through nesting herb-gathering and drying baskets with a glass fairy from Diane Cummings overhead, and a small mirror from Rocio Alarcon between a set of windows to "reflect plant spirits when I see myself."

The consultation room and classroom

Turning right from the front entry is the consultation/teaching room. Above the doorway is a painting of the twenty healers of the Greek Orthodox Church. This was a gift with a holy water blessing included from dear clients. We celebrate inclusion, acceptance, oneness. Deep green wall-to-wall carpeting is soft and inviting. I have many chairs in a circle. One rocker, one overstuffed ample chair, one swivel overstuffed chair, one sofa, a permanent oak massage table with sturdy 4x4 legs, and a long cedar bench along the largest wall. On the bench we set our glasses of water, the medicine kits, and maybe the bag of supplements the client brings. The client sees a painting of a forest scene with a pathway that leads off into the woods. This gives the client an opportunity to let their mind go deeper into the woods of their own thoughts and be able to look to the past and perhaps come up with some memory of whatever their health issue might have been. Or they can sit on the sofa to gaze at an etching of transforming chimes into an Eagle, or see the bay window full of plants and sacred objects, or windows to the street. Plenty of choices. I often light a candle in the line of sight of the client. All are ways to guide the mind, gently, into a deeper space. The client feels nurtured and cared for. I have a throw blanket on the some of the chairs and small pillows here and there. Holding onto something when delving into your personal story is a pretty basic instinct. Security.

I have two medical sheepskins (no arsenic used when tanning). I discovered these when my Mom was dying. They are great for cold people and for floor demonstrations of uterine massage or Yoga. Beautiful Vietnamese baskets for gathering herbs nest in the corner. My past lover Bill donated a glass case to keep my sacred objects, smudging wands, Sweetgrass, Sage, and the basket David Winston's Aunt made. On top of that are smudging items, a ceramic Turtle bowl, Sage jar, and sweetgrass braid. Crystals and sacred objects to hold the energy clear.

There is a sofa that converts to a double bed against the street wall. Plants in the corner.

I don't like to have a desk between my clients and me. I tend to do my intake writing on the back of a book that I hold on my lap. I use Tasha Tudor's *Book of Fairy Tales* because it is pretty, just the right size and weight. It tends to evoke positive responses from clients by adding a subtle element of childish innocence. I use colored copy paper for reminders. These reminders can be the names of herbs, amount of water to consume, therapists to call, foods to buy. I usually write the name of an herb down after it enters my head three times. Confirmation. By the end of the consultation, I usually have a decent formula in progress that I complete in front of the jars in the herb closet or tinctures on the shelves. I also note any issue or herb I might want to get into on the next visit. I copy this paper onto the back of their invoice for the day and hand the original to them.

All around us are some reference books. Some on Ayurvedic diet, wholefood eating: Nourishing Traditions, Staying Healthy with the seasons, The Yoga of Herbs. A book on Acupuncture without needles, a couple of Ayurveda books, Vasant Lad, and one by Candice Cantin.

Beneath that are long, narrow shelves that hold my herbarium box, and two 12x18 herbarium presses. Collecting, arranging, and gluing these earthly beauties to acid-free paper is another form of meditation. Talk about quiet fanatical work! The herbarium box travels with me to lectures in the winter months. I bought 14x20 snap frames, the perfect size to pop a specimen into and take to class. I did make a tapestry carrying case so that the snowflakes and rain wouldn't get under glass. They also make a great addition to herb identification tests for students. Plants are so incredibly beautiful. Under the herbariums are the last of my etching plates, soon to go when the next cleaning frenzy hits.

I have joyously placed all of the Australian Bush Flower Essences plus the entire Flower Essence Repertoire on oak shelves. I have David Dalton's Delta Gardens medicinal flower essences and Kate Gilday and Don Babineau's Woodland Essence's kits of Tree, Bush, Forest Floor, Chakra, and At-Risk essences. And Rhonda Pallas Downey's Path of Wholeness Human Energy System Kit, to draw in the warm dry of Arizona! Flower essences set up a nice vibration in your room. It feels like the entire floral kingdom is on the bleachers just waiting to be called upon, plus you have the vibration of the blessed humans who made these essences.

Into the cupboards I store photo albums of apprentice programs, classes, and conferences. They are large, six photos per page, with room to write above. So far, I have filled seven albums. Great for bringing to lectures or opening to explain what a "medicine show" is. This stopped when digital photography took over. You will only see the younger selves of many now in elder years. Where will they go when I am gone?

Across the room is another bookshelf. *The Flower Essence Repertory, Anatomy, Physiology and Pathophysiology,* and the sixth edition of Barbara Bates's *Guide to Physical Examination and History Taking,* given to me by William LeSassier as his favorite edition, my treasured remembrance and constant source of new insights. Also, a shelf with homeopathic remedies. Away from the energies of people and business. Huna and diagnostic books, Homeopathy volumes and interaction publishing, probably all outdated. Flower essences sit atop the bookshelf away from essential oils.

This room is light and sunny on the darkest of days. I had glass upside-down domes installed where the recessed lighting had been. Subtle etched flowers shining their light on us. I also have a bright full spectrum light I can flip on during dark New England days for facial diagnosis. In order to see each line, color, and marking on anyone's face, decent light is a must. A flashlight will do in a pinch. Remember that bulbs have different hues white, blue, pink. Try to avoid fluorescents and use full spectrum lights.

Off the green room is the bathroom. It's important to keep your bathroom clean. The whole first floor I try to keep immaculately clean all the time. This is public space, and this is professional space. People see that you have a high level of integrity with your cleanliness and make the association with the products you hand them. On the shelves in the bathroom, I keep books on sex, Tantra, aphrodisiacs, sexual abuse, massage and more. People go in there and close the door. If they have a question, they are too shy to ask they might be able to look up the answer. Or the title might trigger an opening to conversation on any one of these subjects. I also like to stay very quiet while they pee so that I gather information about urine power and flow.

Laboratory: tincture preparation room

This room was my acid/etching room when I was a professional artist. My friend painted it deep green; all of it, the ceiling, the floors, the shelves. I wanted it to be a cave, a moss cave to hold the sacred energy of plant medicine. He faux-painted softness onto the walls, ceiling and floor. It looks really mellow. On the walls are some of the plaster "spirit masks" I have created over the years.

The tincture room and laboratory space needs to be immaculately clean. Clients are going to feel more comfortable knowing that you are using sterile jars, and you are making products under sterile conditions. I try to emphasize to my students that their level of cleanliness in the preparation of herbs is extremely important. If you start giving people contaminated product, you are definitely going to get into trouble. When jars are washed make sure the water is hot enough to sterilize (over 220° F). Use a thermometer in boiling water or have a dishwasher with digital settings. Remove paper or plastic linings from lids before washing. Better still, order extra lids so that each jar has a new beginning. Make sure the container is fully dry before capping. Keep caps on jars sitting on shelves. Corks can replace some lids. Rusted lids get recycled. In this room I store tincture preparation jars, wide-mouthed for creating tinctures and narrow-mouthed for storing after the mark

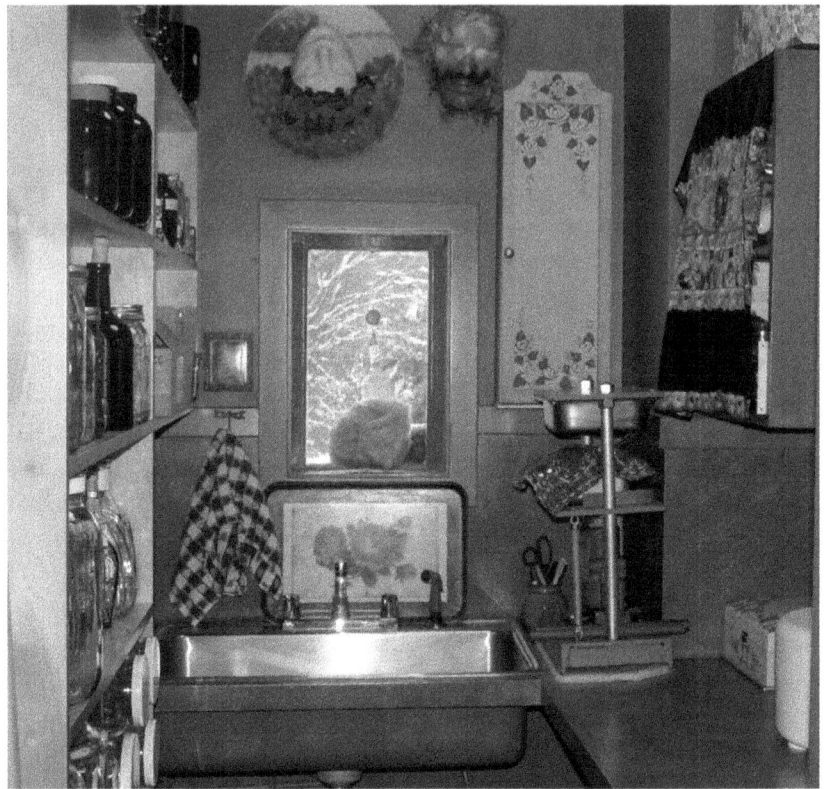

The tincture room

is removed. I have saved corks and keep jar lids in large covered clear-glass containers.

It's best to learn really good habits immediately. Have clean towels everywhere, wash them every day, and wipe down every counter every day. Never use sponges. They are thriving with bacteria after only one use. Use a clean cloth and launder it after one use. I use an Alpine Living Air purifier (they changed their name) with an ionizer to bring down the particulate matter in the air and kill bacteria and viruses. We use a vacuum cleaner with a hepa filter on the floors every single day at the end of the day. In that way the counters stay clean, and the floors stay clean, and it makes people feel more comfortable. I won't say I keep the rest of my house that clean, but I do try.

I have a variable-temperature dehydrator with the dryer on the top. Excalibur Dehydrator. Brilliant. No wet dribbles going into electrical parts! We make lots of dried Nettles, Cornsilk and more. Dehydrated fruits or dehydrated teas are ground to powder for clients.

There is a case each of vodka and brandy constantly being emptied for preparing tinctures. It is wise to keep alcohol under lock and key. Wooden shelves hold the gallon and smaller jars being tinctured. Empty jars await their moment. The herb press is stainless steel and great for getting out every last drop of liquid from the herb. You can teach your clients to make their own products, which is my preference. At this point I don't really have a lot of time to make products, so I prefer to have my clients make their own. Well, that's not true. I prefer they know how to make their own products so that they take their own health in their own hands. As Rosemary Gladstar says, "Herbs are the common man's medicine." I don't have to store their herbal formulas and they are taking responsibility for their own health. They are putting their own energy into their own healing. It's a wonderful way for clients to realize they are in charge of their own health. Teach self-reliance.

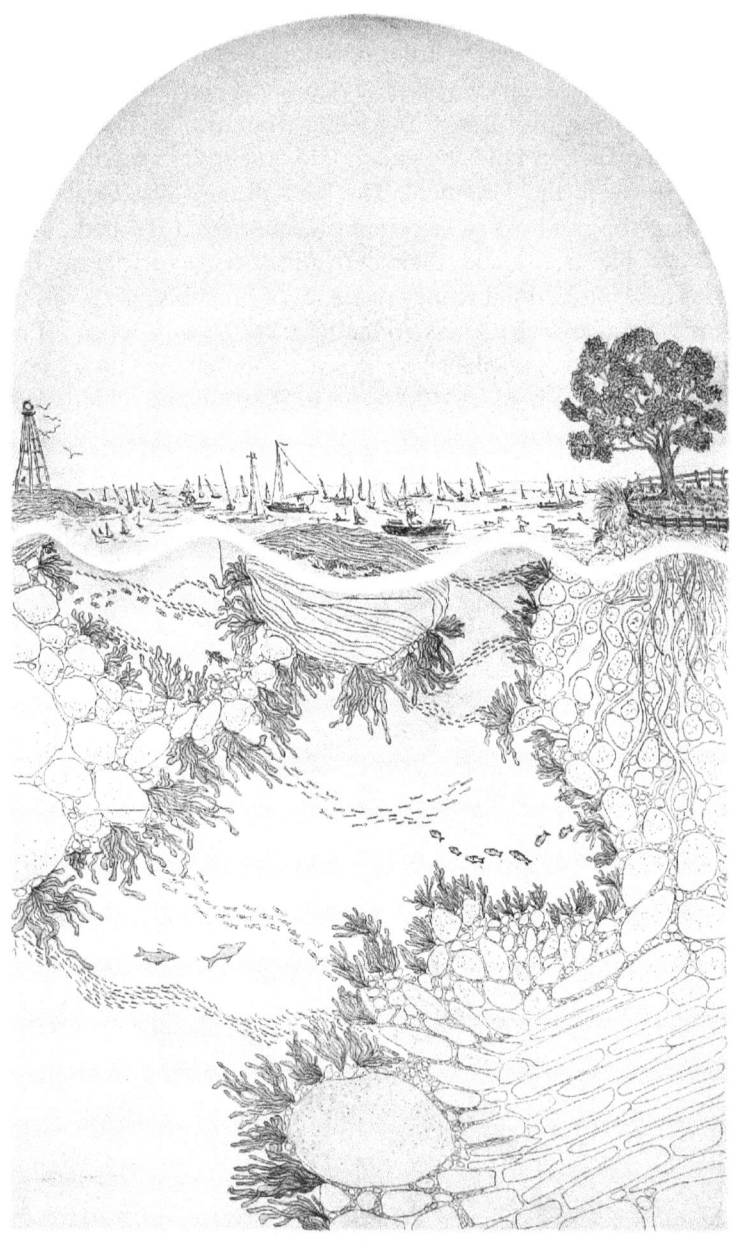

Mid July

CHAPTER 3

Seeing clients

Compliance, identifying the constitutional body types

These descriptions are blended from many classes on Ayurveda, taken with my British friend Anne McIntyre and from Robert Svoboda in his book *Prakriti: Your Ayurvedic Constitution*. Annie explains it quite nicely: "A dosha is a humor, an energy. It's like mind and body physiology. The actual definition is a 'fault' because none of us are born perfectly. We commonly use dosha to mean 'constitution'." If you learn these three body types or doshas, you will be able to formulate for clients more effectively. You will know whether to use herbs in foods, tinctures, teas, baths, steams, or oils. You will have an idea how many times a day a person will actually take something. You will know whether to involve family members in the reminder process. You will know how much of an explanation is needed before compliance is met.

Vata

Vata is air. Air and ether. Vata is the principle of movement. Typical words to describe Vata: Cold, dry, irregular, light, mobile, rough, and insecure. Good tastes for Vata: Sweet, sour, and salty. Bad tastes: Bitter, pungent, and astringent. (Vata is air so these are too drying, which makes Vata emotionally unstable.) Everything about Vata is irregular....

First assure them that being irregular is who they are. To remind a Vata when to take their herbs requires a cell phone timer, or a Pitta to tell them what to do. They are irregular!

Pitta

Pitta is fire. Fire and water. The fire needs food fuel regularly. Pitta is the principle of transformation. Typical words to describe Pitta: Oily, hot, light, intense, fluid, malodorous, liquid, aggressive, compulsive, and sharp. Good tastes for Pitta: Sweet, bitter, and astringent. Bad tastes: Sour, salty, and pungent—too hot. Everything about Pitta is medium....

You need to assure a Pitta that you are smarter than they are. Then they will do whatever you advise.

Kapha

Kapha is water. Water and earth. The principle of substance and cohesion or structure. Typical words to describe Kapha: Cold, wet, and stable; heavy, slow, oily, solid, dense, smooth, and viscous. Good tastes for Kapha: Bitter, pungent, and astringent. Bad tastes: Sweet, sour, and salty. Kaphas have a powerful build and heavy bones, with great physical strength and endurance.

Appeal to the gastronomical pleasures to find compliance with Kaphas.

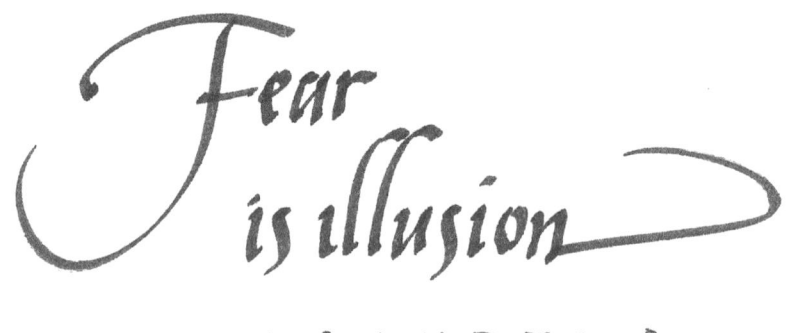

CHAPTER 4

Asking questions

The timeline

This is the most valuable paper to refer to over the following years with a client.

Draw a line mid-way from top to bottom of a blank page. Birth date and birth story at the top. Vaginal birth? Drama? Parents' relationship during those nine months. What were the first words spoken by each parent? Were you planned? Nursed? Atmosphere at home during childhood?

Divide the paper according to their age, in segments of 5 or 10 years. Have their age noted on the left and year on the right. People remember events both by year and age.

Events to place on the Timeline are atmosphere at home, in each living situation, as changes happened, marriages, deaths, separations, divorces, long-term relationships, traumas, dramas, surgeries, accidents, abuse of all kinds, births of children, miscarriages, abortions, vaginal or Cesarian, adoptions, when kids moved out, illnesses, accidents, moving, schools, and jobs.

I use plus and minus symbols next to living situations.

When a client notices that a cluster event happened during a period and an illness appeared they are able to connect and understand the possible cause. Body–mind–spirit are one.

10	1990
15	1995
20	2000
25	2005
30	2010
35	2015
40	2020

Sample of an intake form

As with the rest of this shortened introduction to the hard copy of *The Practicing Herbalist*, there are many stories, recipes, descriptions and further questions after each line of my intake form. Every question has sentences to paragraphs of abundance. Sixty-seven pages more!

Name　　　　**Phone**　　　　**Today's date**　　　　**Address**

Begin a timeline on a separate piece of paper. I add my recommendations on the reverse side.

> *... Our tools work with one of the most powerful forces available the energy of Life or Nature Herself*
>
> M. WOOD

Birth 8/31/1980

Vaginal, home birth, dreamlike, wanted, the scent of roses filled the room

How young are you?

Birth date

Weight

Height

Living situation

What do you hope to achieve with this visit? This is your contract to look back to at the very end.

Any known imbalances

Occupation: Is it toxic? Some jobs are toxic physically, some emotionally. **Like job?** Many jobs are toxic: photography, artwork, dry cleaning, carpentry, painting.... Any previous life exposures to toxins?

Surgeries Note the year and whether other symptoms arrived then.
   Tonsils The immune system's first line of defense.
   Appendix Where the body makes natural biofloras. Ask about constipation. If appendix was removed do they take acidophilus or eat miso regularly?
   Wisdom teeth Temporal mandibular joint problems can begin after having the jaw open a long time. Any teeth cleaning often dumps bacteria systemically.

Taking any medication now?

Supplements? What is the quality, do they break down in water and vinegar? Look for duplications in trace minerals or excess calcium, fillers etc.

What do you do for exercise? Truthfully, by the week. Menopausal women need upper body one-pound wrist weights while walking.

How many glasses of water daily? Half the body weight in ounces is everyone's need for water. There is some water in foods. Coffee takes away four times the amount consumed. Kidneys, blood pressure, and moisture of the entire body are dependent on water. All other drinks are diuretic. Drink with meals? Digestion begins in the mouth. They must add enzymes if drinking all but red wine with meals.

Past or present eating issues? Diets, bingeing, purging. Look to squared-off protruding jaw, acid reflux.

Ages Longer than 3 months is a flag for concern.

Pertinent family medical history Get big issues like mental disorders, heart issues, diabetes, cancer, thyroid issues, on both sides. A family diagram of siblings by age.

Mothers' side, fathers' side Siblings and their health

Current dietary habits

Enjoy your meals? 100 points. **Chew well?** 1,000 points.

Cook own meals? 100 points

How many times a week do you eat?

Fish Essential fatty acids are good. Fried foods are always bad.

Poultry Free range and antibiotic-free?

Red meat Occasional red meats fills the B-12 requirement. Blood type O people may be able to digest meat better than others.

Soy

Mushrooms Are immuno-protective. Not the white button mushrooms, but all others. Shiitake, maitake, oyster, portabella.

Rice, Millet, Barley, Bulghur White, wild, organic? Too much rice without fruit and vegetable fiber may cause rectal prolapse.

Kidney, Black, Pinto beans Beans are full of good estrogens and fiber. Sprout … cook if you are gassy.

Sugar Daily? In what form? White, fructose, honey?

Packaged/frozen food TV dinners? Frozen vegetables?

Salt your food? Table iodized or sea salt?

Vegetables: how many per meal? Suggest three colors daily.

Dairy—organic, small farm?

Raw foods

Fruit Organic? Cherries, strawberries, and grapes are pesticide-rich.

Nuts Pre-soaked almonds and walnuts are protective against cancer. Nuts have healthy fats when fresh. Buy them whole.

Seeds Pumpkin seeds are full of zinc. Men lose lots of their zinc upon ejaculation. Zinc for the dink. People will get white spots on the fingernails have poor tissue integrity and a poor sense of smell when low in zinc.

Miso Healthy bioflora. Rids the body of radiation. Great for city dwellers.

Snacks loved and eaten daily Habits. Comfort foods. Better choices?

Oils used to cook with Olive, small bottles of Sunflower and Avocado cold pressed are best.

Alcohol a week Ask if alcoholism runs in the family: you can get a real strong reaction here. AA works.

Sober? How long? Sobriety is earned through hard work. Congratulate them.

Soda/diet Bubbles are bad for the heart, phosphorous competes for calcium absorption.

Honey Manna from heaven. My Dad is a beekeeper. I am completely prejudiced.

Pasta What type? Non-wheat for skin, respiratory issues.

Caffeine Four cups water for each cup coffee. Chocolate, black tea, green tea.

Baked goods Quality and quantity.

Herb tea Type and consistency.

Eat or drink before bed? What? It is hard to digest foods while sleeping.

Fried foods Including French fries and chips (lose 100 points).

Eat out? Where? What quality of food?

Microwave

Urgent need to eat? Pitta or emotional Kapha. Parasites?

Skip meals? Vata or Kapha.

After eating how do you feel? Bloated, lactose-intolerant?

Drink with meals? Dilutes digestive enzymes.

Cigarettes Heart and lung risk, birth control (if taking birth control pills the hazard is higher). Bone loss. Leaches positive estrogens/testosterone.

Cannabis

Unusual cravings Crave chocolate, need magnesium and calcium.

Are you sexually active? Safely? Happily? Satisfactorily?

AIDS test? Just had relations with virgins? You sleep with every partner your partner has slept with as far as AIDS is concerned.

Enjoy time alone? Get to know yourself first. 1,000 points.

Good social time? Loner? Happy with a few good friends? Lonely or social person?

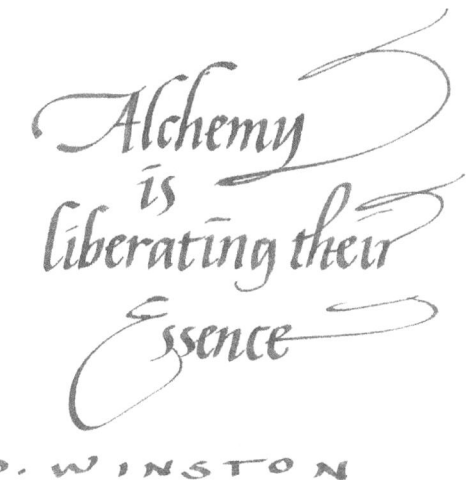

How do you relax? Some people don't know how to relax.

Do you pray or meditate? Great forms of relaxation and focus.

Spiritual path/ higher power/belief in nature? For chronic immune problem.

Belching Lack of digestion

Farting Lack of assimilation, putrefaction, colitis, diverticulitis, spastic colon.

Bowels, describe Urging without results
   Stool slips back, incomplete, prolapsed to vaginal opening. Odor, size, color:
   white—look to colitis
   yellow—look to spleen
   dark—test for blood in stools
   texture—airy or solid
   solid—poor tone, extended transit time or fat malabsorption, add fiber, lower GI deficiency
   irregular, same time daily
   scent
   blood
   mucus
   pain

Abdominal pain Ask them to put their hand on the pain. With visceral pain (pain in organs) you feel the pain when the organ is distended. A broad or diffuse pain. Abdominal pain causes guarding, protective tissues that get ridges.

Liver problems Anger expressed or held in, floaters in eyes, tenderness under ribs, toxin abuse.

Bloating Look to gallbladder.

Gallstones Calcium or oxalate: make dietary changes.

Sore ribs Look to liver, gallbladder, or spleen.

Lump in throat Globus sensation. Teach trachea massage, drink plenty of water. Express emotions. dysphagia, 5th cranial, trigeminal nerve. Check Rx.

Indigestion Do hydrochloric acid test:
Upper GI Deficiency: symptoms are dry mouth, gum and teeth problems, coated tongue, seldom eats breakfast, eats to calm down, indigestion or fullness after eating, slow erratic tone, sometimes has difficulty swallowing, poor coordination of gallbladder, pancreas secretions, fermentation, smelly burps, food sensitivities, use bitter tonics.
Upper GI Excess: symptoms are moist mouth, over-secretion of juices in the presence of food, pointy-tipped tongue which may be sore, seems to eat anything, lots of fat and protein, chronic nausea in the morning or when meal is delayed.

Ulcers Determine which herbs to use.

What makes you happy? Some people don't know; help them find happiness. When have they known happiness in the past?

Bronchitis as a child Scars lungs, years of herbal teas to heal; castor oil packs.

Difficulty breathing Asthma? Allergies? Heart?

Dry cough Moistening herbs.

Base of throat cough Postnasal drip? Adjust the trachea.

Tuberculosis Past family history or exposure.

Congestion Dairy consumption? Allergies?

Wet lungs Osha, check heart.

Asthma/allergies Treat liver; Milk Thistle.

Large bruises Vitamin C deficiency, iron deficiency, leukemia, blood stagnation, fragile capillaries.

Lymphatic swelling/pain Cancer? Mouth sores? Herpes?

How thin were you as a teenager? Bone development is determined then.

Medications taken in childhood Heavy use of antibiotics lead to many problems.

Abused sexually, mentally, physically? Look to thighs and uterus. 2nd chakra. Watch for hesitation or comments like "Well, all kids get hit by their parents." If you were abused, that was a "normal" childhood. Prod gently. Energy work, herbs, and therapy are a great combination.

Constipation Uterine Balancing Class, more water, more fiber, more vegetables, and fruits. Eat meals at the same time daily.

Painful intercourse? Can be a rectocele, prolapse, not enough foreplay.

Hemorrhoids Look to constipation, lack of water, lack of bioflavonoids.

Fissures Look to a hard birthing, constipation, lack of water, lack of bioflavonoids.

Discharge? Color? Consistency? Smell? Time of month? Check for sexually transmitted diseases, candida, fertility.

Onset of menses The later the beginning the lower the chance of cancer. Before age 12 is a higher risk.

Regular as a child? Not unusual to be slightly irregular young.

Regular now? Good endocrine function.

Painful then? Now? How? Cramps, clots, headaches, vomiting.

Painful now? How?

Currently: Days not bleeding 21–30 is the normal range.

Days bleeding 2–5 is normal.

Thin/thick/color Healthy blood is a beautiful red, flowing, and medium consistency.

Heavy ____days Use Yarrow with Cinnamon. Check for fibroids.

Women

Satisfied sexually now? Some people have never really had an orgasm. True.

Low back pain Look to the uterus, kidneys, bladder, financial worries. May start at the feet. Stomach muscles.

Varicose veins Uterine Balancing Class (UBC), more bioflavonoids, Yarrow.

Beginning or end with brown or dark blood? Beginning dark is last month's uterine lining oxidized. Dark blood at the end is lack of uterine tone.

Light days If more than one at beginning or end, more uterine-toning herbs.

Spotting? When? During ovulation? Use a moon calendar to chart any spotting.

Dropped/tipped uterus UBC. Learn to adjust your own uterus.

Heavy feeling above pubic bone? UBC.

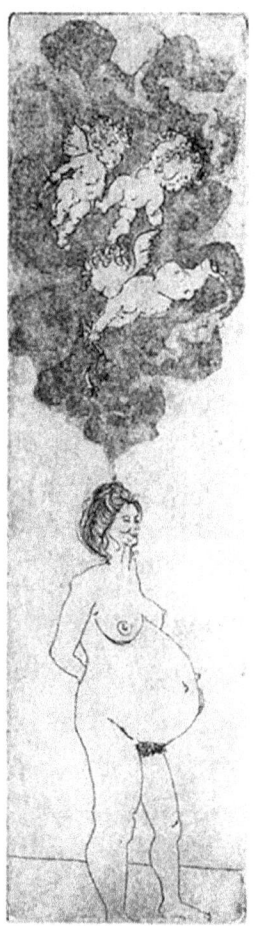

Celestial seeds

Mood swings Amphoteric herbs like Vitex. UBC.

Clotting Too much fibrocystin.

Fibroids Fresh Yarrow tincture is miraculous. Use fairly large doses, 2–3 squirts in water 3–4 times daily.

Cysts Use fresh Yarrow tincture, 2–3 squirts in water three to four times daily.

Tumors Located where? Began when?

Hysterectomy. Why? Ask if they have their ovaries.

#of pregnancies #kids Cesarean/vaginal How was the birth?

Gift? In vitro? Laparoscopy?

Abortions? Miscarriages? Dealt with it? Huge emotional storage if not dealt with.

Pads, tampons, sponge? Bacterial buildup. Commercial pad and tampon products use Clorox/dioxin to whiten, asbestos to cause more bleeding… hmm … do you want that in your private power place?

Birth control used past and present; pills, condoms, cervical cap, IUD, diaphragm, foam, rhythm, lenz.

VD exposure Sometimes there is a residual infection or thought pattern.

Last pap smear? Results? Pap smears should be done the week after bleeding. No penetration during that week so that the cells are not in reaction. They take a bit of the cervix with each sample. How often do you need a pap smear? Cervical cancer in the family?

Raped? I ask this separately from the abuse question. People often say they have not been abused, but "Oh, ya, I was raped in high school." Did they get help? Emotional support? Therapy?

Breasts fibrocystic? Use Yarrow, teach self-breast massage.

Painful? Try Evening Primrose, or the evening primrose.

When? Sore all the time? Add uterine tonics and Vitex. No success, send to the MD.

Surgery: Right or Left A cancer in the right breast is more easily treated.

Lumpectomy/mastectomy/lymph glands How many and where?/**reconstruction/reduction.**

Nipple discharge? Check endocrine function.

Self-exam regularly? Go, girl. Take your breasts into your own hands.

Mammogram? Radiation. Are the breasts painful after testing?

Ultrasound Are the breasts painful after testing? Find another center with kinder technicians.

Menopause? Blood work done?
  Hot flashes? Blue Vervain, Sage spray, cotton clothes and sheets, small fan, vitamin E, EPO.
  Night sweats? Same as above. Chemotherapy hot flashes, night sweats are harder to treat.
  Mood swings? UBC, hormone-balancing herbs.
  Headaches? Look to the liver.
  Bone pain Injury? Lack of minerals? Infection? Hormonal imbalance? Uric acid crystals (gout)?
  Weight gain Thyroid issue? Depression? Lacking Coenzyme Q10? Lethargy?
  Dry vagina Drink water. Add essential fatty acids. Use vaginal lubricants containing Wild Yam or Black Cohosh leaf, St. John's Wort, Calendula flower oils.
  Insomnia how many hours of sleep a night? Lack of sleep can drive a person insane. Eat at normal mealtimes. Workout early in the day.

Name traumatic experiences and when they happened This part of the intake can take quite a while. Some people trivialize their traumas. Some people enlarge them. All traumas have an impact on the whole person. Often a symptom began at the time of the incident. One client recalled being raped as teenager. She had never told anyone before. This experience impacted on many physical expressions in her life. By her making the emotional connections she was able to deal with the body dramas of her past and embrace a pain-free future.

Do you like your body? Create a positive statement.

Cholesterol Eat Oats, raw Garlic and Apples daily. Increase magnesium malate for increased HDL cholesterol. LDLs are "little deadly." In men, zinc will lower LDL levels. Calcium citrate increases the power of the heartbeat. Selenium helps with prostaglandin activity. Coenzyme Q10 is the energy carrier. Brewer's yeast is high in chromium. My favorite teas are Hawthorn, Linden, Rosehips.

Blood pressure Normal is 130/85.

Pain in heart area Muscle tightness. Impending heart attack? Gas?

Poor circulation Cold all the time, invasion of kidneys from extreme cold, bring up thyroid function, sip warm water all day, no liquids in the evening. With eye weakness use Turmeric: do not use with coumadin. Cayenne, Ginger, and Prickly Ash are also good circulatory stimulants.

Cold hands and feet Poor circulation. Raynaud's.

Bruise easily? Iron deficiency or Vitamin C deficiency. Leukemia.

Dizziness? Some endocrine involvement; low BP.

Heart murmur/stroke Look for crooked tongue (stroke). For a murmur use simple heart tonics.

Valves OK? Recommend Echinacea prior to dental work and one week after to protect the heart.

Palpitations Menopausal? Dunk face in ice water. Bugleweed with heart tonics works nicely.

Varicose veins Bioflavonoids. Nodules can form after accidents. Use fresh Yarrow tincture.

Arm pain/jaw pain Signs of heart issues: send to an MD. Women feel like their chin is being pinched when having a heart attack.

Nausea Pregnant? Drugs? Chemo? Food poisoning? Parasites?

Convulsions Alcohol withdrawal?

Stars Pituitary? Thyroid? Low blood pressure?

Fainting Low blood pressure? Anemia? Blood sugar?

Arrhythmia Electrical injury? Mitral valve prolapse? Potassium issue? Did they go off betablockers? My friend Jack did, against my advice, and ended up getting electric paddles.

Cholesterol levels Take Vitamin D, alpha or gamma tocopherol E, 800–1,200 IU. With existing high blood pressure, start low and work up. Eat Oatmeal, Lecithin, Garlic, Guggul.

Swelling hands, feet Edema: drink more water, use Dandelion leaf, Sweet Leaf.

Eruptions Hormonal? Liver related? Lung related? All are digestion related.

Boils Work with improving the condition of the blood.

Allergies Look to the liver, diet, environment.

Asthma Look to the liver, diet, environment.

Dryness Add water, lots of it.

Diabetes?

Itching Add water, lots of it. Bites? Bugs? Poison Ivy? Diabetes?

Hair loss Hormonal? Thyroid? Stress? Dietary lack?

Eczema/Psoriasis Psoriasis on elbow is small intestine or duodenal area: check for.

Discharges from anywhere? Urinary, eyes, nose, ears, outbreaks?

Sleep patterns: wake up at what hour? Adrenals? Blood sugar?

Rapid weight change? Thyroid? Depression? Anorexia, Bulimia.

Headaches: where?
    TMJ—temples.
    Gallbladder—left shoulder tense, up over cranium to left eye.
    Liver—crown.
    Migraine—eyes. Treat the liver. Place cool cloth on forehead, feet in hot water.

Anxiety It feels like… describe symptoms. Use Wood Betony, Milky Oats.

Nervousness In public, private, all the time?

Depression It feels like… Suicidal? Use Kava, they can't jump off the bridge. Use nervine herbs.

Numbness Check cervical spine. Obstruction in circulation?

Fatigue Check thyroid function. Anemia: Floradix, Yellow Dock, Nettles.

Nose bleeds Lack of bioflavonoids. Viral conditions. Nose picking, cut nails.

Use of antibiotics? Look for leaky gut syndrome, too much negative bacteria.

Exposure to genital/oral herpes Use antiviral teas and tincture regularly but rotate formulas.

Foreign travels Look for parasites.

In supportive mental therapies now? Therapy is good, self-therapy is good.

Excessive urination Check for diabetes.

Urinary Tract Infections? History of sexual abuse? Honeymoon syndrome? Menopause? Improper wiping? Wearing pads, tampons after a bowel movement? Knees too close together while peeing?

Ringing ears Use *Monarda fistulosa* for all but bomb and rock n' roll damage.

Water retention Drink more water. Use Dandelion leaf.

Ever been totally cold so you couldn't stop shivering? Kidneys are damaged by excessive cold.

Pee during night? What time? 3:00 am is large intestine; 4:30 is normal renal hormone release time.

Painful urination (before, during, after)

Vaginal warts Antivirals, especially Melissa.

Smelly pee Sweet or sour or strong?

Sediment Look to kidney stones. Herbs. Check diet, uric acid foods.

Thirsty all the time Check for diabetes, too much salty food.

Warm, cold urine Warm is healthy, hot is fever, cold is near death.

Bloody urine Cystitis. Early on use Cranberry capsules or juice. Lots of water. Don't use Cranberry with *Uva ursi*, works best in alkaline urine.

Interstitial cystitis Use probiotics, teas of Cornsilk, Marshmallow, *Uva ursi*, and 3 drops one to three times a day of *Monarda fistulosa*.

Muscle and Joint problems Joints: traveling joint pains are always kidneys.

Backache/upper/lower: which vertebrae? During menses?

Mobility limitations Injury?

Every had a serious fall on your spine? Falling off horses, other moving objects can set up traumas.
   When?
   Where did you fall onto your body?

Broken bones Where? List them.

Spinal curvature Some curvatures can be helped with movement and body work. Refer out to a chiropractor, Rolpher, massage therapist, physical therapist. Use Solomon's Seal or Black Cohosh.

Stiff neck? Structure or tension? Infection?

Sprained tendons/muscles Repeated patterns?

Swollen joints Drink water. Use Turmeric or Wild Yam.

Sciatic pain? Do stomach muscles movements. Strengthen the torso. Use Horsetail.

Loose teeth Mouthwash of Calendula, Prickly Ash, White Oak Bark. Massage the gums.

Failing vision Look to liver.

Failing hearing Look to kidneys and trauma. Use St. John's Wort with Elder to maintain nerve endings.

Gums tender or bleeding Floss, massage, brush teeth. Mouthwash with Myrrh and Propolis.

Sinus congestion Avoid dairy, wheat, corn. Use steaming herbs. Use essential oils topically (Chamomile, Lavender, Melissa).

Sinus infection Avoid dairy, wheat, corn. Steaming herbs, Goldenseal capsules, Echinacea and Eyebright tincture—at least ten days straight.

Sore throat Avoid dairy, wheat, corn. Echinacea tincture. Gargle with sea salt and warm water. Lemon juice and honey drinks.

Ear aches Avoid dairy, wheat, corn. Keep them covered. Too noisy at home? Use herbs above.

Eye pains dry/wet, floaters More water, but not near food. Use alteratives: Dandelion, Burdock, Red Clover with Cleavers or Calendula.

Hay fever Avoid dairy, wheat, corn. Use Goldenrod tincture and Milk Thistle seed.

Back of knees hurt Stagnation, use liver tonics and lymphatic movers.

Lower body symptoms Liver symptom.

Varicose veins? Constipation? Lack of bioflavanoids? Lack of exercise?

Big vein on side of head when lying down Use Nettles.

Name two emotions dominant in your life now, … and… What are the corresponding organs?

Men

Up to pee at night Teach Kegels. Intake of fluids before bed?

Fertility issue Swingy not clingy underwear. Add 800 IU of Vitamin E. No Cannabis. Add zinc (pumpkin seeds). Eat lots of seeds, nuts, eggs, and other fertility-rich foods. Use pelvic tonics.

In the service? Where? Each war had its own unique poison.

Nocturnal emissions This is unusual in adults, may have a deeper issue at hand.

Premature ejaculation Use Schizandra berry daily. Read books on Tantra and holding the semen.

Incontinence Teach Kegel exercises. Causes: injury, infection, obstruction, stones, tumors, drugs (diuretics), removal of prostate.

Drippy after urination See above—early stages. VD.

VD exposure When and where?

Abused mentally/physically/sexually Look to thighs and prostate. 2nd chakra. Watch for hesitation or readjustment of his body in the chair. Prod gently. Oh, you were brought up… parents. Oh ya, a little slapping around…. Hmm. The Priest got too friendly. Your Uncle was drunk…. All abuse issues need to be told (if not to you to a therapist) and released. Energy work, herbs, and therapy are a great combination. The Bush Flower Essence Fringed Violet with Little Flannel Flower.

Jock rot Clean clothes daily. Herbal powders.

Kidney stones Calcium or uric? Eat Apples daily. Drink plenty of water. Boiling down the emotions?

Impotent Use Prickly Ash, Panax Ginseng, Ho Shu Wu, Schizandra, Ashwaganda.

Sit all day Get off that prostate! Same goes for bicycles.

Prostate checked lately? Good idea.

Testicles swelling/lumps Use lymphatic drainers (Calendula, Cleavers, Burdock). Refer out to MD.

Painful Use poultices of Chamomile, Ginger, Calendula. Refer to MD.

Anything unusual or causing difficulties?

Describe your birth

Family problems impacting on your life now? Family has a huge impact.

Describe any pains not covered… And the direction it goes… What causes it?

Are you affected by weather changes? Full spectrum lights are great for Seasonal Affective Disorder. Walk at noon. Don't wear photosensitive glasses.

Anything I missed?

Write down your physical observations: Pulses (Vata, Pitta, Kapha). Appearance of nails, skin, tongue coating and color with a drawing of distinguishing lines on tongue, ears, face. What is the tone of voice? What is the temperature of hands? Take a digital photo for the file.

What are your expectations for resolving your present health problems? Have them make a positive statement about improved health.

What participation are you willing to take? Teas, pills, tinctures, capsules, syrups, routine exercise, everything. Dietary changes? Make an agreement how to follow the protocol. How many times daily? For how many weeks or months?

With all intakes the major headings can be generally addressed. Especially if one aspect is pressing. You may return to any of these sections in the next session. Be sure to note this for "Next time."

Hand over your invoice, looking them in the eyes, smile on your face, for this excellent exchange of sharing. Receive money with gratitude. The investment in your career, and belief in the plants, now supports you.

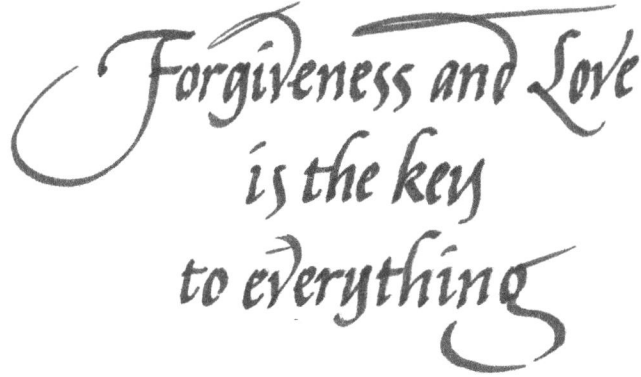

Forgiveness and Love is the key to everything

—KARYN SANDERS

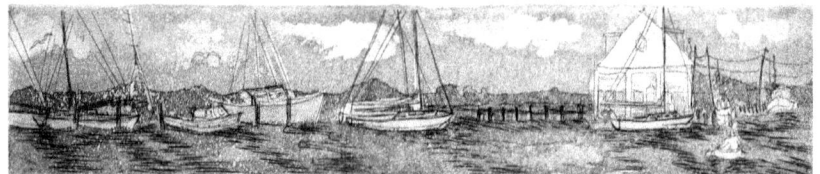

Islanders

CHAPTER 5

Understanding the endocrine cascade

I thank my teachers, especially Tammi Sweet, for being such an amazing Anatomy and Physiology teacher. I know I have simplified and left out way too much, oh well. I also honor Phyllis D. Light, Kate Gilday, Christa Sinadinos, Matt Wood, and Ian White for all your wisdom.

    The endocrine system is the magical cycling and recycling of vital energy in the form of hormones, enzymes, coenzymes which we call vitamins, minerals, and the building blocks of the human body—amino acids. This dance from glands at the top of the cranium to the pelvic floor glands defines a great deal of how we feel as we walk this amazing planet Earth. I have found that having a basic understanding of the endocrine cascade, noting which gland may be out of synch, or undernourished, or overstimulated helps my clients regain homeostasis. Whatever it is that has made them feel "less-than" and out of balance, unhappy, infertile, or stunted in some growth pattern can be remedied. Be it physical or emotional, knowing the indicators and potential solutions gives us clues to nourish the endocrine system into transforming in a good way.

    Here are three simple tips. One: Good nutrition is necessary for endocrine health. "The only way to change your DNA is with food.

In order to receive the white light of your potential you must eat well," says Jeff Bland. Two: You might consider keeping your cellphone way away from all those endocrine glands. Texting is safer. Three: Keep in mind that the liver must be healthy in order to properly process the hormones passing through.

Hormone is from the Greek *hormon*, "to urge, to urge on, impulse." Hormones are made from cholesterol; progesterone, estrogen, testosterone (androgen), aldosterone (mineralocorticoids), and cortisol (glucocorticoids). Cholesterol is also the precursor for Vitamin D, the material making up the membranes of cells, and the insulating membranes of myelin in our nervous system. Vitamin D levels have plummeted across the lands. Bile acids are synthesized in the liver from cholesterol and secreted in bile. Yes, we need cholesterol! It courses through our blood between the liver and all other tissue. So keep your liver healthy.

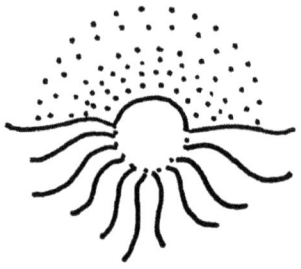

Pineal gland

Circadian rhythms, night and day, happy and sad, reproduction, self-recognition, immune health. The cycles of life. The precursor hormone is the neurotransmitter serotonin from L-tryptophan.

The pineal gland is between the eyes, two fingers up into the forehead, right where the Hindu bindi (circular mark) is placed, and toward the center of the cranium. It sits between the two halves of the brain communicating with the cerebrospinal fluid. It is cone- or mushroom-shaped and described as the "Third Eye." The balance and interplay of light and dark, within the soul and outside the body, the feelings of sadness and happiness, the undulating circadian rhythms are the manifestation of life ever-changing in the pineal gland. This is truly the "enlightenment" receiver.

UNDERSTANDING THE ENDOCRINE CASCADE 67

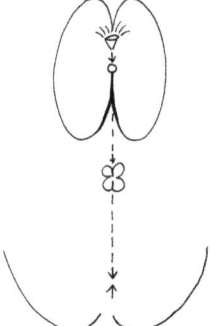

Pineal to reproductive and basic emotional foundation

The hormone produced by the pineal is melatonin, which eventually deals with pigmentation of the skin. "The pineal sits like a lotus with the cerebrospinal fluid flowing beneath and through it. As we age we produce less melatonin, and tan less from the legs upward. It is like the lighthouse beacon releasing signals in response to body changes," shares Tammi Sweet. Melatonin is stimulated by Darkness and inhibited by Light.

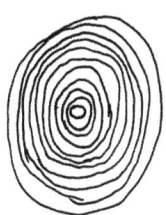

Pineal rings

The pineal accumulates brain sand or pineal sand with age, which is "radioplaque calcium phosphate" and carbonate granules, which can be seen in X-ray. We are like trees: our rings are in the pineal gland and these rings show our age! This sand is radioactive, or EMF (electromagnetic field) sensitive and responsive, and is affected by the magnetic changes of our Earth's magnetic rings. Does the pineal also tune into the magnetic fields of other life forms? Yes, I believe it does. When I was studying Polarity Therapy, we energy receivers would notice bizarre shifts, odd, rolling movements or balance changes in our bodies that corresponded to magnetic field changes around this planet. Some ring around the Earth had shifted. Earthquakes. "Parathyroid functioning plays a role in the sand-layering process," Tammi Sweet intones.

Melatonin is derived from L-tryptophan and serotonin released into circulation immediately upon synthesis. It is so important to have a darkened bedroom as light inhibits melatonin production. Being human we are meant to walk and exercise in daylight, let the light in, and sleep in the very dark, be in deep rest, allowing the secretion of lots of melatonin.

No LED lights from clocks computers or cell phones. Remove them from the room entirely, cover smoke detector lights with tape, and block windows well with shades or curtains. Nicole Telkes says: "Nine PM is when the pineal gland turns on—no light when sleeping!" Even though you sleep, your eyelids see through to the light. Control over the secretion of melatonin is maintained by nerve pathways from the retina in the eye that provides self-regulation of circadian timing by the suprachiasmatic nucleus (SCN) complex. This promotes certain restorative and anabolic processes such as core temperature regulation, sleep patterns, cardiovascular output, antioxidant function, and anticancer activities as well as interaction with reproductive function. Kathleen Maier says: "If you are exhausted in the day you possibly don't have enough energy to sleep. Sleep requires good sound energy."

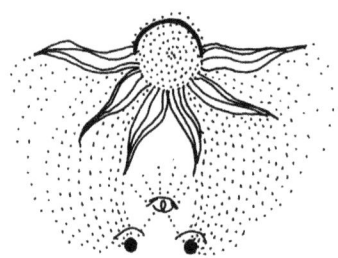

Serotonin is a neurotransmitter that carries information across the synapse between one neuron and another. It is found in the brain, gut, pineal gland, and blood vessels; it causes blood vessels to narrow, reduces aggression, affects color pigmentation via melatonin, affects mood, emotion, sleep, appetite metabolite 5-HTP (excitotoxins also use 5-HTP receptors), and helps reduce pain.

Somewhere in here is a connection to the amygdala. Our amygdala has to do hormonal secretions relating to the emotions of fear, anger, arousal, and pleasure from past and present memories and motivations. On my "timeline" these are the events with the greatest weight. Memory and emotions are combined in the amygdala, so traumas such as being beaten, abused, or degraded are stored in the cellular memory. DMT, Dimethyltryptamine, under extraordinary circumstances, is also produced by the pineal gland. Birth, some mushrooms and extreme emotions push the pineal to create DMT. Just as powerful stimuli are positive combinations of memory and emotion—being loved, accepted, cared for, and praised. Many extremes can be favorable. Here I interject words from Kathleen Maier: "The pineal gland is about transformation and transition." This is where the moan comes in. "Orgasm is the little death—our egos dissolve and we give ourselves over to unite with the divine."

Meditation helps to bring balance to the endocrine glands. If you don't formally meditate, meditate informally. Light a candle, sit comfortably with spine erect at the table and stare at the candle. After a minute or so shut your eyes, and bingo! The light shines on your third eye. After a few minutes of letting the thoughts pass through your mind like clouds, get up and you have done a good thing for your stress level and endocrine system.

Environmental pollution, poor nutrition, high altitude, stress patterns, and a blow to the head also impact the pineal gland. Cold water hitting the back of the neck keeps you younger by stimulating your core temperature regulatory center. Avoid fluoride; it accumulates in the pineal gland.

Visual indications for the pineal gland

- Darkened nipples during pregnancy.
- Dark vertical line of the pregnant belly.
- Eye sand, where the Sandman leaves grit in the morning.
- Dark circles under the eyes.
- Pigment changes circling the lips, splotches on the face.
- Pigment changes anywhere on the skin.

Other indications for the pineal gland

- History of a blow to the head.
  Madeline, a 15-year-old soccer star (endocrine-damaging sport), was hit in the forehead, hit the back of her head and had her forehead hit once more during the same impact play. Sent to the bench and home.

The concussion was discovered when her parents took her to ER. Madeline went from active honor student to Sleeping Beauty, sleeping 18 hours daily. She was unable to stay awake for more than a few hours at a time. This had been going on for a year. She had a history of bone issues, calcaneonavicular coalition (birth defect, lack of intrinsic factor) and shin splints, had constant pain and a red-tipped tongue (heat in heart/thyroid).

I gave her an Oatstraw decoction (40–50-minute simmer) adding St. John's Wort aerial parts, Hawthorn flower and leaf, and Hibiscus flowers to infuse. 3 cups daily. Drops of Rosewater into drinking water. Tincture of Sweet Leaf, *Monarda fistulosa*, Yarrow, Skullcap (8 drops daily). tincture of Black Cohosh, Solomon's Seal, and Arnica, 4 drops daily. Spray of White Sage for muscle pain (as needed). Her improvement was phenomenal. Was it because so many of her herbs treated endocrine as well as lack of intrinsic factor deficiencies? Madeline is now in school full time and earned membership into the National Honor Society.

- Cryptococcus neoformans (parasite of central nervous system), Huntington's disease, Optic neuritis, Parkinson's, Multiple sclerosis, PKU, Spina bifida, etc.... all are possibly connected to a lack of melanin.
- Lack of natural light reaching the eyes.
- Wearing contact lenses, eyeglasses that have Ultra Violet block.
- Working unusual shifts, nights working, days sleeping.
- Radiation exposure.
- Poor sense of direction.
- Magnetic field changes.
- Temperature swings.
- High altitude.
- The gastrointestinal tract secretes melatonin and serotonin. Are gut instincts poor?
- Jet lag.
- SAD (seasonal affective disorder).
- Depression.
- Autism.
- Cancer, including breast cancer.
- Breathing irregularities.
- Insomnia.
- Multiple sclerosis.

- Epilepsy.
- Exposure to fluoride.
- Fear of orgasm.

Nutrition for the pineal gland

Make sure you have abundant L-tryptophan and serotonin to create melatonin. Tryptophan is an essential amino acid that is needed for the production of niacin, serotonin, and melatonin. The body cannot produce tryptophan, so it is essential that you get enough from your food.

- Bone broth.
- Watermelon and pumpkin seeds, seaweeds, and dairy products.
- Legumes: lentils, fava beans and other beans, chickpeas, dairy—yogurt, milk, cheese.
- Protein foods: beef, pork, turkey, chicken, fish, shellfish, eggs—most especially lightly cooked egg yolks for D3 to balance cortisol.
- Whole grains: oats, brown rice, wheat, wheat germ.
- Nuts and seeds: hazelnuts, peanuts, almonds, sunflower seeds.
- Chocolate—yes.
- Consume *less* caffeine, nicotine, alcohol, high doses of B-12, beta-blockers, calcium-channel blockers, NSAIDs, and SSRIs.

www.solawakening.com has some cool meditations and images to play with.

Herbs for the pineal gland

- Passion Flower aerial parts.
- St. John's Wort aerial parts.
- Motherwort aerial parts.
- Valerian root.
- Blue–green algae.
- Medicinal mushrooms.
- Mints aerial parts.
- Blue Vervain aerial parts.
- Sassafras inner bark.
- Hops strobiles.
- Nettle leaf.

- Sarsaparilla bark.
- Wood Betony aerial parts—if gut instincts are poor.
- "Eastern Skunk Cabbage flower essence—purple flower is the shape of an inverted pineal gland," shares Sean Donahue.
- Australian Bush Flower Essence "Bush Iris," 7 drops twice daily.
- Woodland Essence Chakra Essence "Crown" knowing. Day and night light and dark, Quieting. 4 drops twice daily.

Supplements for the pineal gland

- Amino acids L-tyrosine, and L-dopamine, L-tryptophan (do not use if taking Rx SSRI, MAO inhibitors). MAO inhibitors block chemicals that break down serotonin tricyclic antidepressants—prevent breakdown of serotonin, dopamine, and norepinephrine.
- B vitamins, niacin. Sublingual with intrinsic factor deficiency.

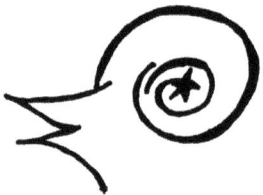

Hypothalamus: "the master gland"

Keep in mind that the liver must be healthy in order to properly process the hormones passing through it.

Hypo means "under," so the hypothalamus is under the thalamus. It is all about barriers, boundaries, and homeostasis, which is ultimately the goal of herbal practice. With the pituitary it creates and pulses life-sustaining, life-altering amino acids through the bloodstream. Amino acids are the building blocks of the body.

Within the cranium is the amazing mixture of glands and brain parts that keep us functioning. Sensory data pours into our thalamus, which sends it to our amygdala. We process it both through our thinking mind and through our store of past fear responses. (These are actually two different processes—if our trauma response is activated our conscious decision-making process is bypassed.) And in less than a second, signals are sent throughout our body through our nervous system. All intertwined with messages to all the endocrine glands via the hypothalamus.

When we look at a side view of the cranium the thalamus, amygdala, and hypothalamus create the head of a bird with the furthest back point being the pituitary. The master gland—master of what? Yes, all the hormonal instruction and perhaps more than that, the focal point of light brought in by the pineal gland, dispersed to the other endocrine glands, which may be enhanced by meditation and mind-full focus.

The hypothalamus is the gland that expresses and directly deals with stress through control of the pituitary. It is hard, and silly to try and separate the results and functions of the hypothalamus, pituitary, and adrenals. The HPA Axis is the interplay between these three stress-responding glands. The hypothalamus controls our flight-or-fight response by releasing hormone signals to the pituitary or autonomic nervous system. Neural information is transformed into hormonal information. Magic. Hormones from the hypothalamus all end with RF for "releasing factor." Remember that factor means hormone. The hormones are released to the anterior or posterior pituitary. Cortisol levels increase under stress. When the HPA Axis is suppressed, we become depressed.

For many years, the pituitary gland was called the "master" endocrine gland because it secretes several hormones that control other endocrine glands. We now know that the pituitary gland itself has a master—the hypothalamus. This small region of the brain below the thalamus is the major link between the nervous and endocrine systems. (It also ties into memory and emotion responses from the amygdala.) It receives input from the limbic system, cerebral cortex, thalamus, and reticular activating system. It also takes in sensory signals from internal organs and from the retina. Painful, stressful, and emotional experiences all cause changes in hypothalamic activity. In turn, the hypothalamus controls the autonomic nervous system and regulates body temperature, thirst, hunger, sexual behavior, and defense reactions such as fear and rage. This master gland is about the size of a cherry.

I had a client who had constant head injuries. He also played soccer and hit the ball or the ball hit him constantly. He became depressed, could not sleep and made decisions without realizing the long-term consequences. All of his symptoms led me to endocrine disruption.

The hypothalamus is an important regulatory center in the nervous system as well as a crucial endocrine gland. Cells in the hypothalamus synthesize at least nine different hormones, and the pituitary gland secretes seven. Together, these sixteen hormones play important roles in the regulation of virtually all aspects of growth, development, metabolism, and homeostasis. The hypothalamic hormones are an important link between the nervous and endocrine systems.[1]

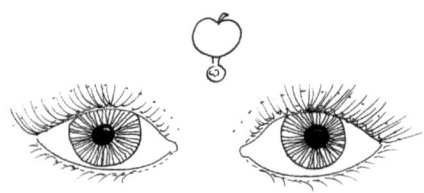

The posterior pituitary is not separate from but an extension of the hypothalamus. It hangs down as a stalk from the pituitary. Oxytocin (maternal and sexual bonding, ejection of milk, uterine contractions) and the anti-diuretic hormone vasopressin are produced in the posterior pituitary. It is the vascular connections between the hypothalamus and pituitary that are crucial. That is why blows to the head have such a damaging effect. The anterior pituitary is developed separately in utero; it secretes protein hormones.

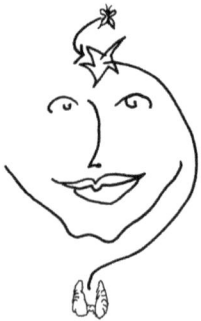

The hypothalamus produces spurts of hormones into the blood as it flows to the pituitary. Thytrophin releasing hormone (TRH) when it

---

[1] Tortora, G.J. and Derrickson, B. Principles of Anatomy and Physiology, 11th ed. (Wiley and Sons, 2006), p. 625.

gets to the pituitary produces thyroid stimulating hormone (TSH), and prolactin (PRL), a protein of 198 amino acids—wow, powerful milk.

Gonadotrophin releasing hormone (GnRH) is a peptide of ten amino acids that is all about sexual physiology. It secretes every couple of hours, causing follicle stimulating hormone (FSL), and

luteinizing hormone (LH) maintains the corpus luteum, releasing estrogen and progesterone in females, and testosterone to go up in males.

Growth hormone releasing hormone (GHRH) is two peptides (polypeptides are chains of amino acids made of one or more polypeptide molecules) with over 80 amino acids stimulating cells in the anterior pituitary to secrete growth hormone.

Corticotrophin releasing hormone (CRH) is a peptide of 41 amino acids released from the anterior pituitary to release adrenocorticotropic hormone (ACTH). ACTH is a peptide of 39 amino acids acting on cells of the adrenal cortex to stimulate production of cortisol (glucocorticoids—the conversion of fat and hormones into glucose), the steroid aldosterone (mineralocorticoids—responsible for mineral metabolism, reabsorption of sodium into the blood, water follows the salt and maintains normal blood pressure), when at normal levels (when produced in excess elevates blood pressure by favoring retention of excess sodium, changing the volume of blood in the system), and androgens (male sex hormones—testosterone).

Somatostatin is a peptide of 14 amino acids and one of 28. This one inhibits the release of GH and TSH. It is also released in the pancreas and intestine where it inhibits other hormones. GH in the pituitary promotes growth by binding to receptors on the surface of liver cells. Then they release IGF-1—long bone growth.

Dopamine is a derivative of the amino acid tyrosine. It inhibits prolactin (PRL). Prolactin, a protein of 198 amino acids made in the pituitary, promotes milk production, and synthesis of milk. It is stimulated by TRH and repressed by estrogen and dopamine.

Ask: "Did you ever have a blow to the head? Play soccer?" Frequent blows to the head often affect the hypothalamus, pineal, and pituitary in a bad way.

Visual indications for the hypothalamus

- Tripping constantly over the same threshold, carpet, or tree root in the path.
- Unusually thin—look to anorexia nervosa (too much GnRH) or bulimia.
- Hyperthyroid or hypothyroid—test for Eleuthero root or Pulsatilla flower.
- Blue–black circles under the eyes.

Other indications for the hypothalamus

- Addictive behaviors like abundant eating, tobacco, alcohol, sexual dysfunctions, too much sex or "mattress dancing," as Phyllis D. Light says, drugs (pharmaceutical and recreational), computer and other screens, and excess working.
- Attention deficit disorder (ADD)—Look for distraction from task, tipping back in chairs, laying head down on arms at the table, one eye "lazy," food allergies. Test for Eleuthero or Pulsatilla.
- Short-term memory issues.
- Temperature irregularities from hot to cold and back again. Test for Eleuthero or Pulsatilla.
- Inconsistent emotions. Test for Eleuthero or Pulsatilla.
- Lack of a sense of consequences for actions.
- Bipolar, manic depressive behavior: Blue Vervain (tension above), test EPA/DHA.
- Cushing's syndrome (high cortisol, adrenal hormones) (tumor) or from therapy for rheumatoid arthritis.
- Anxiety. Test Passion Flower.
- Erotomania, fetishes (posterior pituitary): Blue Vervain (tension above).
- Obsessive-compulsive behavior (posterior pituitary): Blue Vervain (tension above).
- Post traumatic stress disorder (PTSD).
- Chronic fatigue and fibromyalgia, other autoimmune disorders.
- Irritable bowel syndrome (IBS). Test Shepherd's Purse, Slippery Elm.
- Frontal headache during menses and pregnancy.
- Crave dairy, have high prolactin levels that suppress other hormones—gain weight. Stop milk products. Test Wild Carrot.

- Partners who do not remain monogamous—look to the posterior pituitary, vasopressin and oxytocin deficiency. Excessive sex and not bonding.
- Losing fluids—urine, premature ejaculation, leukorrhea (posterior pituitary). Test Schizandra, Shepherd's Purse.
- Pee all the time (vasopressin) at night: bladder or prostate (take glycine).
- Polycystic ovaries (LH anterior pituitary).

Nutritional support for the hypothalamus

- Gobo (Burdock root).
- Thiamine-rich foods B-1—Sunflower seeds, fruits and vegetables, split peas, whole grains, bran, lima beans.
- B-12 rich foods—fish, red meat, mollusks, turkey, crustacea, eggs.
- Vitamin C—citrus fruits, Red Bell Peppers, Potatoes, Strawberries, and Cantaloupe.

Herbs for the hypothalamus

- Burdock root. Burdock is for the big strong person who collapses from within. This is bear medicine that makes you strong and leads you to the other medicinal herbs you need. It also reestablishes pre-flora and intrinsic factor that is missing from the gut with ADD, and many other "disorders." Isn't a dis-order really a deficiency of some essential nutrient?
- Passion Flower aerial parts. The flower looks like it came from outer space. The color of the crown chakra, it treats all of the upper four endocrine glands. It is wild and reaches out in wiggly tendrils on vines, wanting to connect and circle round anything nearby. Passion Flower reconnects you with the healthy sleep cycle, hormone cycles, and earth cycles.
- Arnica flower is for trauma. Arnica from the Colorado Mountains is especially potent. Nicole Telkes is an ethical wildcrafter who makes primo extracts.
- Red Clover aerial parts. Oh, gorgeous clumps of purple to red blossoms, bursting upward, shaped as a head, or cranium meeting at the neck to send and receive vital hormonal information from sky to earth. Leaves with the chevron triune, maiden–mother–crone, letting us know she is for all transitions of life through all life.

- American Ginseng "Man root", for that man root, or woman root as the case may be. Another five-finger plant saying "Come to me" or "Go away." This plant truly speaks to vital energizing of we humans. This plant is the grandfather of all plants and is our biggest adrenal booster. Red berry, great mover of blood and growing deep in the forest and hard to find—use it with respect.
- Schizandra. This potent antioxidant berry has five tastes—sweet, sour, salty, pungent, and bitter. It is for all issues of fluids letting go at the wrong time. Urine, semen, tears.
- Woodland Essence Flower Essences 6th and 7th Chakra Essences (Throat and Knowing). 4 drops twice daily.
- Australian Bush Flower Essence Bush Fuchsia. 7 drops twice daily.

Supplements for the hypothalamus
- Sublingual B-12.

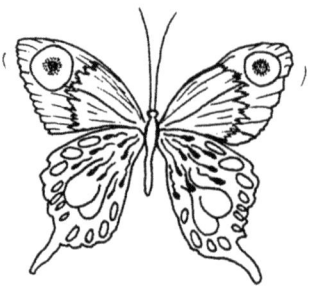

Pituitary gland

The pituitary is below the optic nerve in a butterfly-shaped bone (Sella turcica) connected to the hypothalamus through a stem of vascular networks. The pituitary deals with growth hormone (GH), fat and glucose metabolism, bone growth, and protein metabolism, RNA formation (ribonucleic acid: single- stranded molecules transcribed from DNA in the cell nucleus or mitochondrion or chloroplast, substituting the sugar ribose for deoxyribose, the nucleotide base uracil for thymine), stimulates digestion, and also effects immune function. Levels of GH are increased by amphetamines, estrogens (including Soy, Cannabis, and Hops), Parkinson's medication (Levodopa), and B-6. Corticosteroids can give a false normal in blood tests. Nervous system depressants (chlorpromazine—psychotropic drugs) may suppress GH.

Thyroid stimulating hormone (TSH) or thyotrophin, a glycoprotein, consists of a beta chain of 118 amino acids. It has an alpha chain of 92 amino acids identical to FSH and LH and chorionic gonadotropin. It is this beta chain that makes TSH special. We know that being special has its own price to pay.

Secretion of TSH is stimulated by arrival of thyotrophin releasing hormone (TRH) and inhibited by arrival of somatostatin from the hypothalamus. TSH stimulates the thyroid gland to make T4. Hyperthyroidism is the body making too many antibodies against their TSH receptors—Graves' disease. A deficiency of TSH causes hypothyroidism. Low TSH may lead to osteoporosis.

Follicle stimulating hormone (FSH) is the same alpha chain in TSH and LH and a beta chain of 118 amino acids. It is stimulated by GnRH and highest in women days 1–14 mid-cycle and menopause. In men it stimulates sperm development.

The intermediate pituitary works with melanocyte stimulating hormone (MSH), pigmentation—ah, back to the pineal gland. Look to the pineal herbs.

Ask about causes of pituitary imbalance: stress, birth control pills or hormone replacement therapy, radiation exposure, blows to the head, growths or tumors, surgery, malnutrition, and loss of blood supply.

Visual indications for the pituitary

- Pituitary pimple. Around ovulation a large volcano-like pimple that does not come to a head, above the left ear about 2 finger-widths up.
- Short but normally proportioned child.
- Dwarfism (growth retardation from not responding to GH from genetic mutations).
- Gigantism (hypersecretion of GH).
- Acromegaly (hypersecretion of GH or GHRH).
- Crease in the ear lobe—high blood pressure from too much ADH, collapsed capillary bed.
- Long arms and legs.
- Goiter.

- Cretinism.
- Slow tooth growth.
- Skin darkening—Addison's disease.

Other indicators for the pituitary

- Peripheral stars in line of vision.
- Dark exudate from nipples.
- Rapid weight gain or loss, 7–10 pounds.
- Fainting.
- Polycystic ovary syndrome.
- Inflammation and bloating. The pituitary gland is related to stomach issues.
- Cushing's disease (hypersecretion of ACTH—too much cortisol for too long). Look for a fatty hump between the shoulders, rounded face, and pink/purple stretch marks.
- Hard belly—cortisol reaction.
- High blood pressure from ADH.
- Hypopituitarism by tumor, infection or injury, or restricted blood supply.
- Lack of sexual characteristics—I have seen this in Kauai. GMO experimentation, unknown by the public for years, this continued genetically engineered testing genetically affected all life on a small island.
- Decreased sex drive.
- Small penis growth—look to pesticide, BPA, GMO foods in the diet or fertilizer exposure disrupting the endocrine system.

Nutritional support for the pituitary

- Avoid corticosteroid medications.

Herbs for the pituitary

- Sumac tips are for losing fluids of any kind. Sumac contains fluids good for ADH issues, diabetes, etc.
- Burdock root.
- Vitex berry is the herb to bring back hormonal balance in women, relieve post-partum depression, and regulate the menstrual cycle.

- Yellow Cowslip Orchid Australian Bush Flower Essence. 7 drops twice daily.
- 7th Chakra, third eye, ability to be conscious. Woodland Essence. 4 drops twice daily.

Supplements for the pituitary

- Taurine for neurological health, d-phenalalanine, L-tyrosine (a precursor to neurotransmitters tyrosine, then dopa, then norepinephrine, then epinephrine), L-tryptophan for sleep. Take between meals.

A note on ADH (anti-diuretic hormone) blood tests—False high readings if pregnant, consuming diuretics, Licorice, progesterone or if you exercise just prior to the test. False low results from a low salt diet. Remember to suggest raw salt—it is many minerals, not sodium alone.

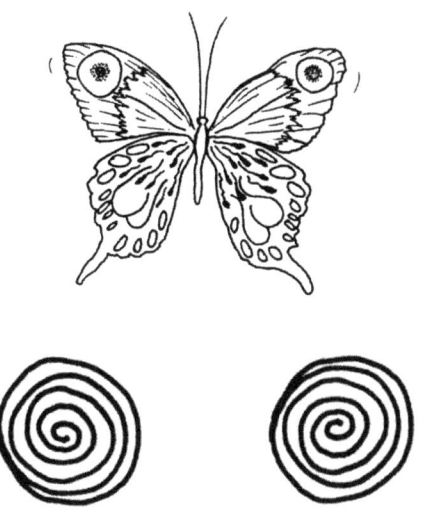

Adrenal glands

The adrenals sit atop the kidneys. The outer layer is the adrenal cortex, which surrounds the adrenal medulla. Adrenals are a part of our sympathetic nervous system. "Eat, enjoy and relax," says Tammi Sweet. Vata people can't eat when stressed. They work with the hypothalamus and pituitary by producing releasing hormones to hormones that stimulate the adrenal glands. A cascade. Adrenal exhaustion is easy to see. The issues causing stress must be directly faced. Ask: "What do you and don't you have control over?" Begin by encouraging, pointing out the one thing the person does control. Start by changing that. Even when they are tired they must move daily. Begin with a ten-minute walk and slowly increase the time. Walk inside buildings when weather is slippery or too hot or cold.

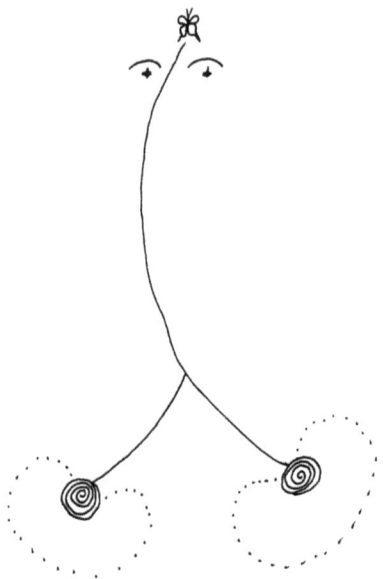

The **adrenal cortex** (outer region) has to do with metabolism, chemicals in the blood, and body characteristics. The adrenal cortex produces:

Hydrocortisone (Cortisol) dealing with fats, proteins, and carbohydrates. Lowest at midnight, highest production 6:00 am.

Corticosterone with hydrocotisone suppresses inflammatory reactions and affects the immune system.

Aldosterone helps maintain electrolyte balance by how much salt and water is excreted in urine, which regulates blood volume and pressure.

Androgenic steroids are converted to male (androgens) or female (estrogens) hormones (Androgen hormones) in the testes or ovaries.

All these hormones affect the body's use of fats, proteins, and carbohydrates.

The adrenal medulla (inner region) produces norepinephrine and epinephrine (adrenaline), helping us to deal with stress.

UNDERSTANDING THE ENDOCRINE CASCADE

Epinephrine (adrenaline) "I'm scared!" Adrenaline deals with stress by increasing the heart rate and force of contractions, takes blood flow from the digestive organs to the muscles and brain, relaxes smooth muscles, converts glycogen to glucose in the liver and lets you RUN.

Norepinephrine (noradrenalin) has vasoconstrictive effects—so it increases blood pressure.

Visual indications for adrenals

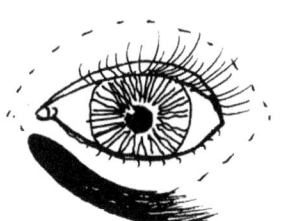

- Swelling abdomen (cortisol reaction, adrenal excess). Blood sugar will be high, the person slowly gains weight and has a cortisol squirt right after allergic food is eaten (hard belly), usually gluten, casein, eggs, sugar, soy, corn. M.W.
- Blue–black circles beneath the eyes.
- Diagonal line in the ear lobe.
- Gray colorations in skin, eyes, and tongue.
- Tremor of tongue and hands extended.
- Irritability.
- Dilating and contracting pupils.
- Fingernails with ridges.
- Poor digestion, indigestion, food allergies.
- Tongue white coating.
- Anemia.
- Lazy white blood cells.
- Muscle spasms, facial twitches.
- Skin tags (high cortisol), undigested proteins.
- Baldness (hyperandrogenic).
- Shortness.
- Boys who grow quickly young, slow down too young (hyperandrogenic).
- Acne (hyperandrogenic).
- Girls with fused labia, masculine genitalia (hypoandrogenic).
- Hirsutism—hair growth on the face and body (hyperandrogenic).
- Breasts become smaller.
- Small penis (hypoandrogenic).
- Small testes (hypoandrogenic).
- Urethra opening malformed.
- Inflamed and red, pitta, "Clint Eastwood—A lean, mean fighting machine."
- Inflamed digestion, Kapha-bear type.

Other indications for adrenals

- Light-headedness upon standing (hypoaldosterone).
- Low blood pressure (hypotension) (hypoaldosterone): too much sodium in urine, increased potassium.
- Inflammatory conditions (high cortisol).
- Immune suppression, autoimmune issues (high cortisol).
- Insomnia.
- Weepiness, unsure of life's path.
- Hormonal irregularities.
- Exhaustion.
- Osteopinia, osteoporosis (high cortisol).
- Weakness.
- Low libido (high cortisol).
- Increased libido (hyperandrogen).
- Heart disease.
- Infertility (high cortisol).
- Brain fog.
- Constipation.
- High cholesterol (high cortisol).
- High blood pressure (high cortisol).
- Polycystic ovary syndrome.
- Girls miss menstruation, puberty (hypoandrogen).
- Deep voice (hyperandrogen).
- Uterus shrinking (hyperandrogen).

Nutrition for the adrenals

- Sleep!
- Fish.
- Flax seeds and oil (fresh).

No caffeine, artificial sweeteners, and flavors.

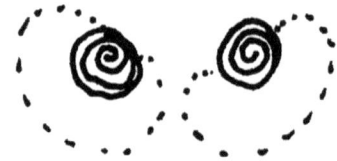

Herbs for the adrenals

- Licorice is so valuable for endocrine health, is demulcent, relaxing and healing to exhausted adrenals, and protects the liver. Cool. When I suggest Licorice many people express aversion. This is usually from eating sugary fake strings of candy when young. Give them a sample and see if they change their mind. It reduces Pitta—inflammation and gas are lowered.
- St John's Wort aerial parts.
- Ginger root.
- Chickweed aerial parts. Succulent ground cover, Chickweed is a great herb to reduce masses, your total mass or lypomas, fatty or other cysts.
- American Ginseng root will give an energetic lift, and just a little bit goes a long way. Ginseng assists blood sugar imbalance, immune, digestive, circulatory, and nervous systems.
- Black Walnut hull.
- Red Pepper fruit.
- Fo ti.
- Milk Thistle seed.
- Flax seed.
- Saw Palmetto berry.
- Raspberry leaf.
- Eleuthero root (hyperadrenal).
- 1st Chakra Safety and Security, 3rd Chakra Self, Will and Power Woodland Essence. 4 drops twice daily.
- Macrocarpa Australian Bush Essence. 7 drops twice daily.

Supplements for the adrenals

- Dietary enzymes to help with production of cortisol and aldosterone.
- Systemic enzymes if there is scar tissue, PCOS.
- Evening Primrose Oil.
- Fish Oil EPA-DHA.
- Magnesium.

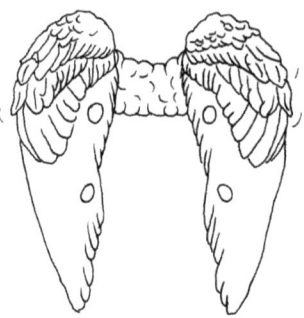

Thyroid gland

Ask: "Have you been in an accident where your neck was jerked? Whiplash? Seatbelt across your neck? Have a job using cleaners? Surgery near the thyroid where it was moved aside? Anesthesia? Changed your diet radically? Exposed to radiation—live by the ocean, on granite, in a city, on planet Earth?"

Treat the upper endocrine gland's symptoms first, pineal, hypothalamus, and pituitary. Do remember the endocrine system is a magical system of creation and connection, cycling and recycling!

General indications for the thyroid

The thyroid reflexes to metabolism, the eyes, eyebrows, neck, hair, and nails, and leads to other endocrine disruption, testosterone low. The general feeling is exhaustion, not getting enough oxygen, weight gain or loss, obsessive-compulsive behavior, depression, and sleep issues, apnea, and mitral valve problems. Every organ depends on thyroid hormones.

When the thyroid is not functioning well a person will have hot or cold sensitivity, autoimmune issues, and headaches. The person tends to be very intuitive. They may have orthostatic hypotension (light-headed when getting up to stand from lying or sometimes even sitting). People with thyroid conditions have a propensity to calcify, creating bone spurs and hardening of arteries. Vitamin D is critical to osteoblast (bone) formation.

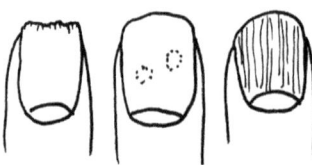

Meditation for the thyroid

Meditation can reinvigorate the thyroid. Sit comfortably, stare at a lighted candle and then shut your eyes, envision the sun shining above your head and allow it to funnel into the crown and flow out through the "third eye" (the point between the eyebrows two fingers above, where the bindi dot is placed on people from India). Just two minutes a day of this simple light work will assist all endocrine glands.

General nutritional protection for the thyroid

With three indications of imbalance begin nutritional shifts. When you catch it early enough, ten years before it shows up on the blood test, you can really do a lot of work with food. If taking thyroid medication, be careful how much Kelp is eaten. The iodine levels have to be well monitored. There are different types of seaweed, each with a different level of iodine. Use raw, untreated, unchanged sea salt instead of iodized table salt. Milk is a source of iodine that affects all people. Every commercial teat in the USA is dipped in iodine, and not the iodine that is helpful to our endocrine glands.

When you support adrenal function, sometimes thyroid issues clear up.

Testing for the thyroid

- "When the back of the neck is open the thyroid opens," explains Karyn Sanders. I ask the client: "What feels better, tipping your head forward or backward?" Hypothyroid imbalance feels better backward, hyperthyroid feels better forward.
- Hit ankle nerve on Achilles tendon: strong reflex is hyperthyroid, low reflex is hypothyroid.
- Paint iodine, the size of a quarter, on to inner arm between elbow and wrist. If it is absorbed quickly you need iodine, and if slowly you don't. Iodine is in sea vegetables, apricots, eggs, blackstrap molasses (also rich in potassium and calcium). The Eclectics used potassium iodine for enlarged spleen and cerebral vascular insufficiency.
- See visual indicators listed.
- Basal metabolic rate for men and women. Use a non-mercury glass thermometer; shake it down the night before. Sleep alone, in a

non-latex, non-heated bed, blankets and PJs covered normally. Moving as little as possible, place the thermometer in armpit, leave there for 10 minutes. Auxiliary body temperature should be between 96.8° and 97.6° Fahrenheit. Do not test during menses or ovulation. Chart for at least 3–5 days. Below 97.6° F may indicate hypothyroid.
- Last we turn to blood tests. I have found that thyroid issues don't show on blood work until the issue has been lived with for ten to fifteen years. Levels of thyroid stimulating hormone (TSH)—this is produced by the pituitary, and generates T4 production, low TSH leads to atrophy. A low TSH (0.5) is important in thyroid cancer, since TSH levels promote thyroid cancer.
T4: Poor T4 function: two things to implement: 4, 5, 6 drops of iodine, coupled with tyrosine. See if basal body temp goes up.
Free T4.
T3 has to do with growth and development.
Free T3.
R (reverse) T3.
Thyroid globulin level (can be used to assess thyroid cancer and autoimmune thyroid conditions).
T peroxidase (also to assess thyroid cancer).
DHEA blood test. If you support adrenal function, sometimes thyroid issues clear up. Low levels of DHEA contribute to inadequate conversion of T4 to T3. In some people, if there's a lack of harmony and communication, they will make more estrogen.

People with low aldosterone, low blood pressure, get dizzy easily, pee frequently, usually need salt, and benefit from licorice. A solid extract of Licorice, a little salt, in some saturated fat (coconut water) works well here. Deer antler extract, a Ginseng, and an adaptogenic plant.

Thyroid cancer is often radiation-induced: check carcinoma embryonic antigen, thyroid globulin and calcitonin levels (elevated) in thyroid cancer.

T3, free T3, and RT3 are most important markers. You want to see a good, high level of T3, and a low level of RT3. Stress induces the RT3 to go up. Lots of cortisol in the adrenals will make T4 turn into too much RT3, because the body wants to slow the metabolic rate and keep some reserve.

Remember, all of the endocrine glands cycle together. If you support adrenal function, sometimes thyroid issues clear up. Be sure that the pineal, pituitary, and hypothalamus are functioning well. Phyllis D.

Light plans to publish her book on the endocrine system soon. She has been a great inspiration to me.

Environmental impacts for the thyroid

Ask: "Have you been in a car accident or had a blow to the neck?" The seat belt may have hit the thyroid gland at impact. Surgery in the area of the neck, especially if the trachea is moved, can temporarily harm the thyroid or parathyroid. Many prescription drugs lower thyroid function, including birth control pills.

Look at the bigger picture as well: what surrounds the person? A coal plant (mercury), plastics in drinking bottles, pipes, storage containers, clothing? Dangerous cleaning products?

I feel that triclosan in the environmental is especially a culprit here. I have had a number of clients reverse this diagnosis when they remove toxins from their home and employ the benefits of herbs and energy work. "How to avoid triclosan—forgo antibacterial soap: The American Medical Association says not to use it at home. Watch for triclosan (and triclocarban) in personal care products: Read ingredient labels or use Skin Deep to find products free of triclosan and triclocarban, its chemical cousin. Avoid 'antibacterial' products: Triclosan is used in everyday products."

These include toothbrushes, toys, and cutting boards that may be labeled "antibacterial," or make claims such as "odor-fighting" or "keeps food fresher, longer." Triclosan may be in these products: It's nearly ubiquitous in liquid hand soap and dishwashing detergent, and towels, mattresses, sponges, personal care products, shower curtains, toothbrushes, phones, kitchenware, and plastic food containers, shoes, flooring and carpets, clothing, fabrics, and toys. A U.S. FDA advisory committee has found that household use of antibacterial products provides no benefits over plain soap and water, and the American Medical Association recommends that triclosan not be used in the home, as it may encourage bacterial resistance to antibiotics. "Triclosan is linked to liver and inhalation toxicity, and low levels of triclosan may disrupt thyroid function," according to the Environmental Working Group, EWG.com.

Exposure to too much iodine from cold and flu and heart medications, especially lithium, and contrast dies for X-rays may fill the body with toxic levels of iodine. If you add some iodized salt shaken on to foods daily and the body rebels.

Fluoride in water depresses thyroid function. I have a whole house filter plus a Reverse Osmosis filter on the drinking water.

> Live on planet Earth? Nuclear power plant leaks emit radiation which affects this entire round planet. Radiation falls down with the rain on to your lovely head. The nuclear power plants all create risk, as proven by the failure of Fukushima. Granite-rich lands and cities hold radon and emit radon gas. Be sure to cover the thyroid when having dental, or any X-rays. Thyroid cancer is often radiation induced: Check carcinoma embryonic antigen, thyroid globulin and calcitonin levels (elevated) in thyroid cancer.

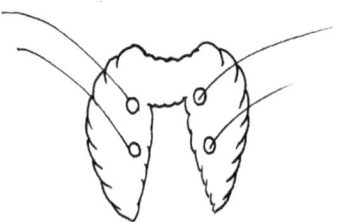

Parathyroid gland

The parathyroid secretes parathyroid hormone (PTH), increasing calcium in the blood from our bones, or reabsorbed from fluid in the kidneys or from contents in the small intestine (calcitriol, the active form of D). It also regulates the level of phosphate in the blood. Make sure there is ample hydrochloric acid in the stomach!

Matthew Wood says the parathyroid type is the "Rabbit Family," "Prince Charles, needing nutrition."

Visual indicators for parathyroid

- Hair loss.
- Muscle spasms.
- Cataracts.
- Edema.
- Nervousness, twitchy.
- Fine bones.
- Medium height.

Other indicators for parathyroid

- Low calcium.
- Tetany (involuntary contraction of muscles).
- Muscle spasms.
- Vomiting.
- Diarrhea.
- Nerve pain.
- Headaches.
- Abdominal pain.
- Hyperparathyroidism tumors in the parathyroid, raising blood calcium levels, weakening bones.
- Hypoparathyroidism from damage during neck surgery, PTH gene family history, family history of autoimmune attack of parathyroid (DiGeorge syndrome).

Nutrition for parathyroid

- Green leafy cooked vegetables: Collard, Turnip, Mustard Greens, Bok Choy.
- Blackstrap molasses.
- Cooked Broccoli.
- Okra.
- Nut milks, nut butters, Sesame seeds, Tahini.

Absolutely no cola drinks! They suck too much calcium from the bones!

Herbs for parathyroid

- Wild Yam root.
- Nettle leaf.
- Horsetail aerial parts.

Supplements for parathyroid

- D3 calcitrol.
- CalApitite from bone.

Hyperparathyroid (high)

Indications for hyperparathyroid

- Itchy skin (calcification or red blood cell death).
- Depression.
- Exhaustion.
- Confusion.
- Kidney stones.
- Diarrhea.
- Abdominal pain.
- Excess urination.
- Aches and pains.
- Nausea.
- Headache.
- Green cast to skin.
- Joint pain in fingers.
- Abdominal groans.
- Psychosis.

Nutrition for hyperparathyroid

- Blackstrap molasses.
- Raw salt.
- Water.

Herbs for hyperparathyroid

• Skullcap aerial parts.	• Mullein leaf and flower.
• Passion Flower aerial parts.	• Yellow Dock root.
• Blue Vervain aerial parts.	• Dandelion leaf.
• Sassafras root	• Horsetail aerial parts.
• Mushrooms fruiting body, mycelium.	• Lady's Slipper: endangered, use sparingly.
• Chickweed.	• Sea vegetables.

Supplements for hyperparathyroid

- Multi-mineral.
- Less Vitamin A, D, dairy, calcium, iron.

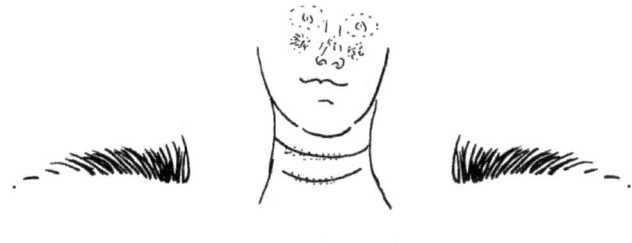

Hypothyroid

Visual indications for hypothyroid

- Thinning outer eyebrows (also parathyroid).
- Hair loss—especially mid to outer eyebrows (clumps of hair falling out may be pituitary or hypothalamus); sparse hair on forearms or lower legs (also parathyroid).
- Ring lines above and below the thyroid ringing the neck.
- Skin, hair, and nails are dry and brittle.
- Edema, face and body look puffy, can't hold onto water, non-pitting in lower legs.
- Weight gain shows as a big belly and abundant thighs. Try Bladderwrack or Chickweed for obesity.
- Vertical ridges on nails indicate digestion is poor.
- Eyes lose their shine.
- Eyelids droop over eyeball.
- Little scratches heal slowly.
- Broken capillaries on nose and cheeks. Ruddy or rosy complexion, including around the mouth.
- Walking with palms facing backward.
- A "big white pasty tongue," says Matt Wood.
- Tendency to pallor, especially around mouth. In dark skin, it darkens around mouth, forehead, and sides of face.
- Goiter, enlargement of the thyroid gland, is quite easy to see from afar. *Iris versicolor* helps a sluggish liver, very specific for goiter or enlarged spleen.
- Dark shadows, puffiness or sunken under the eyes.
- Bruising easily indicates possible iron depletion.
- Pigment distribution (use pineal gland herbs). Vitiligo—white spots or patches on skin.

Other indications for hypothyroid

- Metabolism is slow.
- Body temperature is cold, hands and feet are cold.
- Voice is deepened or gravelly.
- Constipation.
- Snoring may occur.
- Depression.
- Food allergies causing inflammation.
- Cysts and growths on the thyroid. Low iodine, hyper- or hypothyroidism, cyst or tumor. Use Red Root.
- Headaches.
- Foggy thinking.
- Cholesterol and triglyceride may be high.
- Libido may be low.
- Irregular periods and heavier bleeding during cycles.
- Infertility.
- Miscarriages. I have many clients who had frequent miscarriages until the thyroid was nourished. Metabolism of hormones is bad, look to the liver.
- Tired but can't sleep.
- Apnea or shallow breathing. Low oxygen and breathing issues, and being susceptible to every respiratory bug that passes by.
- Calcium deficiency indications: Bone spurs, arthritis, lost or cavity-filled teeth, degenerating vertebrae, osteopenia, osteoporosis, and insomnia.
- Low stomach acid contributes to the lack of calcium assimilation. Yes, foul scents emerging from the body.
- Hashimoto's thyroiditis is considered autoimmune, where the body attacks the thyroid. Plenty of Rosemary. "Pitta run amuck," M.W. (parathyroid)

Nutrition for hypothyroid

Eat *more*

- Yams, Sweet Potatoes, carotenoid-rich foods.
- Walnuts.
- Black beans (specific for adrenal and thyroid connected).
- Parsley.

- Strawberries.
- Apricots.
- Sea vegetables; Kelp, Bladderwrack and Hijiki. A piece of Kelp the size of your little finger daily with lots of water.
- Sesame seeds are great, Tahini also good. Make Gomasio—sesame seeds and sea salt with kelp to grind on to foods.
- Oats for sleep and nervous system support. I love Milky Oats or a long decoction of Oatstraw.
- Almonds.
- Bananas.
- Olive oil improves thyroid function.
- The amino acid tyrosine is created by the thyroid—so feed it Carob, cooked Oats, Mustard Greens, Spinach, Pumpkin seeds, Cabbage, Snow Peas, Butternut Squash.
- EFAs are rich in glutathione foods. Avocados are a perfect food.
- Royal Jelly promotes fertility (with Saw Palmetto).
- Selenium-rich foods (as long as soil contains it) are Brazil nuts, Garlic, Onions, and Russet Potatoes.

Eat *less* Peaches, Pears, Beans, and Soy, cruciferous vegetables: including Broccoli, Cabbage, Brussels sprouts, Cauliflower, Kale, Spinach, Turnips, and Mustard Greens unless cooked. Carbohydrates are a common food allergy when in the form of bread, bagels, and other baked goods or "bads." Do avoid commercial dairy products for at least three months and keep refined carbohydrate consumption and sugar to a minimum.

Herbs for hypothyroid include

- Sea vegetables including Bladderwrack, Kelp, and Hijiki contain soluble iodine. This is what Kelp does:
  "Kelp grows out of the primordial waters of the ocean telling me that it is both an ancient and a divine healer. The fact that it looks like a hand with fingers makes me think of the hand of creation. Its deep rhizoids remind me of an umbilical cord. The blades and fingers remind me of healing hands that welcome an opportunity to become nurtured and reconnected to the spirit of the Divine. The little gas-filled bladders remind me of little life preservers. Kelp can not only heal the human body and deliver hormone stimulation; it does the

same thing for other plants. It provides oxygen and a healing and nurturing environment for other forms of sea and land life. It is both the hand and womb of creation. The color of Kelp reminds me of the color of stagnation. Kelp is a mucilage demulcent. It helps to move lymph fluid and works on the gastrointestinal system. It prevents fat from building up in the cells and removes environmental and metabolic toxins."

"Kelp makes the hormones, the little messengers, work better. It is a plant of communication, whether it's teaching our bodies how to communicate or connecting us to the ocean's floor. It affects my thyroid which is located in my throat, the home of my voice box, and the third chakra. As a fitness instructor and fitness instructor, my calling is to communicate physical awareness to others. By adding Kelp into my daily life I have a feeling that I will be able to call on the ancient and Divine qualities of its signatures, thus allowing the will and power of the universe to work alongside my observations.

"I don't think that there is a place on earth unaffected by the pollution caused by man. Thank God for the rejuvenating and restorative powers of seaweed." Deb Wilczek, from her report at North Shore Community College.

- Gotu Kola aerial parts.
- Chickweed aerial parts. Chickweed is a great herb to reduce masses, your total mass or lipomas, fatty or other cysts.
- American Ginseng root will give an energetic lift, and just a little bit goes a long way. Ginseng assists blood sugar imbalance, and the immune, digestive, circulatory, and nervous systems.
- Sarsaparilla bark.
- Parsley aerial parts.
- Burdock root.
- Ashwaganda root—I like this for the nervous system and feeling "strong as a stallion."
- Oats aerial parts.
- Coleus—an Ayurvedic herb that improves thyroid function and glycolisis, and normalizes gene expression.
- Gotu Kola aerial parts. Gotu Kola is my favorite "too much thinking" Vata nervine, which may increase thyroid hormone and decrease dryness and brittleness.

- Vitex berry is hormonal regulation for the hot times, the maidens with irregular cycles and volatile airs, kicking in endocrine regularity for reproduction frustrations, hormonal calming for adolescent boys as their scent and primal desires peak. Amphoteric. Brings to balance higher and lower chakras.
- Passion Flower is also a favorite before bed. It is especially for people who awaken between 2:00 and 4:00 am "wired and tired."
- Blue Flag.
- Wild Carrot seed (Queen Anne's Lace).
- Saffron stamen improves oxygenation in the body and is antidepressant.
- Also include Cinnamon, Ginger, and Cayenne to stimulate metabolism.
- Licorice is so valuable for endocrine health, is demulcent, relaxing, and healing to exhausted adrenals, and protects the liver. Cool. When I suggest Licorice many people express aversion. This is usually from eating sugary fake strings of candy when young. Give them a sample and see if they change their mind. It reduces Pitta; inflammation and gas are lowered.
- Rosemary. Plenty of Rosemary in cooking. Rosemary helps gene transcription. Karnasol, a phenolic compound in Rosemary, is good for thyroid, and for regulating autoimmune thyroid conditions. Compounds in rosemary modulate oxidative stress in the body. Another compound in Rosemary is hydroxytyrosol, and with the karnasol it scavenges oxidative damage. In CO_2 extracted Rosemary essential oil you get lots of phenolic compounds.
- Old Man Banksia Test for Australian Bush Essence of Old Man Banksia. 7 drops twice daily.
- 4th Chakra Woodland Essence. Throat, speaking your truth, communicating honestly and clearly. Also hypothalamus, what we choose to do and the consequences of choices. 4 drops twice daily.
- Christa Sinadinos has published an excellent book, *The Essential Guide to Western Botanical Medicine*. Go to it for detailed descriptions of thyroid herbs including those already listed and Schizandra, Devil's Club, Spikenard, Elk Clover, California Spikenard, Reishi Mushroom, Rehmannia, Oregon Grape, Milk Thistle, Turmeric, Yellow Dock root, Ginkgo, Hawthorn, and more.
- Avoid teas containing Lemon Balm leaf and Blue Vervain leaf, in more than occasional amounts.

"Drop doses of fresh plant extract of Pulsatilla 3–5 drops 3x day: Indications: melancholy, sadness, poor circulation, open and week pulse, reproductive imbalances and a tendency to weep easily." (Donald Yance sees this profile a lot with thyroid and breast cancer.)

Supplements for hypothyroid

- Selenium is very important. Fifty percent of the public is deficient in selenium, because our soil is low in this mineral. Chlorine depletes selenium; make sure your water is chlorine-free. When gardens are watered, selenium is depleted, and ultimately the vegetables are deficient in selenium. Selenium is a critical co-factor in glutathione production, and for converting T4 to T3. We all may benefit by taking 200 mcg selenium.
- Test for supplements of magnesium, potassium, calcium, Vitamins A, D, E, C, B-multi, D3, E, and zinc.
- The amino acid D-phenylalanine taken between meals in loading doses can stimulate more thyroid production of tyrosine. Don't take amino acids if melanoma is present or when taking SSRIs.

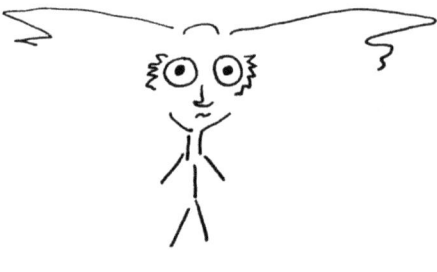

Hyperthyroid

Hyperthyroidism is the production of too much thyroid hormone. An overactive thyroid usually swings. Herbs are great because they harmonize.

Visual indications for hyperthyroid

- Bulging eyeballs.
- High-pitched voice.
- Decrease in weight.

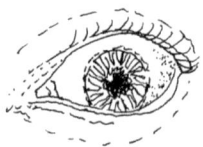

- Inability to gain weight.
- Hyperactivity.
- Goiter.
- Tip of tongue with vertical columns. Kay Parent adds: "A vertical indent just above the tip of the tongue, which is clearly visible which seems to indicate a stress on the thyroid. It precedes test markers, but can appear alone or with other diagnostic indicators."
- Graves' disease is increased thyroid hormone.
- Toxic adenomas are nodules on the gland then secreting thyroid hormone; a goiter may appear containing several nodules.
- Subacute thyroiditis is inflammation of the thyroid gland, usually a short-term issue.
- Pituitary gland issues or tumors in the thyroid gland. If pituitary, ask about seeing peripheral stars, a pimple in the hairline above the ear at the line of the eye, nipple exudates, and fainting. Medical testing is advised.

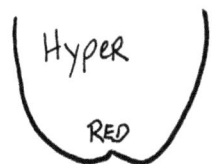

Matthew Wood shares: "They have the look of a hunted animal, a nervous hasty manner, with red complexion and tongue, a rapid, hasty pulse, sometimes with nervousness, wakefulness, sleeplessness, nervous fear, anxiety, restlessness, and high sugar consumption, with swelling of the lower calves."

Nutrition for hyperthyroid

These foods should be *included* in the diet for hyperthyroid conditions as they depress thyroid activity:

- Cruciferous vegetables: including Broccoli, Cabbage, Brussels Sprouts, Cauliflower. Drink Cabbage juice, immediately after juicing.
- Leafy greens: Kale, Spinach, Mustard Greens.

- Turnips.
- Fruits—Peaches, Pears.
- Beans.
- Soy (if you believe it is GMO-free).
- Flax seeds—Raw Flax crackers and fresh, refrigerated Flax seed oil, 1,000 to 15,000 mg daily.
- Avoid dairy, wheat, alcohol, and caffeine products for at least three months.

Herbs for hyperthyroid

- Motherwort aerial parts. She makes you float. The seedpods are satellite orbs, prickly and beautiful, green leaves with jagged, irregular edges like irregular heartbeats. She is the perfect three o'clock in the afternoon fix for the busy person. Instantly calming.
- Bugleweed aerial parts.
- Lemon Balm aerial parts. Hyperthyroid.
- Chickweed. M.W., P.D.L.
- Black Walnut hull. M.W., P.D.L.
- Licorice root can help build up DHEA. Licorice is a precursor to estrogen, progesterone, glucocorticol hormones, and adrenal hormone. Licorice is also highly anti-carcinogenic.
- Passion Flower, aerial parts, is also a favorite before bed. It is especially for people who awaken between 2:00 and 4:00 am "wired and tired."
- Old Man Banksia Test for Australian Bush Essence. 7 drops twice daily.

Kay Parent has successfully used David Hoffmann's formula: Tinctures of Bugelweed 4 parts, Motherwort 2 parts, Skullcap 2 parts, Hawthorn 1 part. One dropper three times daily, or thrice daily when across the pond.

Supplements for hyperthyroid

- Vitamin B complex with extra riboflavin (B-2) and thiamine (B-1) and B-6 (pyridoxine) 50 mg, 3 times daily with meals. Vitamin B injections may be necessary. Brewer's yeast 1–3 tbsp daily: it is rich in many Bs. If deficient in intrinsic factor use sublingual or shots of Bs.

- Essential fatty acids (EFAs) as directed on label; it is needed for correct glandular function.
- Lecithin in soft-boiled eggs aids in digestion of fats and protects the lining of all cells and organs.
- Vitamin C in fruits or supplements is important in this stressful condition.
- Vitamin E 400 IU daily, no more. This may stimulate the thyroid gland; however, a small amount is needed.
- Calcium and magnesium help many metabolic processes function correctly. Calcium and magnesium must be present together in sufficient quantities, or the body can't use either. The optimal ratio is 3 parts calcium to 1 part magnesium. Never supplement calcium without also supplementing magnesium, because if you do so, the body will actually use its stored Mg to try and process the supplemented Ca, the end result of which is that the body actually depletes its stored calcium reserves because the magnesium holding it in place was taken away in trying to process the supplemented calcium. If you think about it, all the extra calcium added to foods and drinks these days only results in us having lower calcium levels overall—due to the magnesium not being supplemented… not good, not good at all! So, if you supplement Ca, make sure to supplement 1/3 as much Mg at the same time. 1,000 mg of Ca needs 334 mgs of Mg; 1,500 mgs of Ca needs 500 mgs of Mg.

If you really want to suck the calcium out of your bones and teeth, drink the well-known colas.

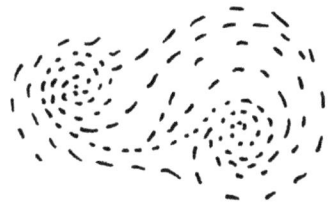

Pancreas

The pancreas is blended exocrine (squirts into ducts) and endocrine gland. It is about assimilating this world we live in. The pancreas has a tail touching the spleen, and endocrine tissue secreting insulin (a hormone that controls the amount of sugar in the blood) and glucagon (a polypeptide hormone secreted in response to a fall in insulin) internally and pancreatic juice externally into the intestine.

The greater mass of the pancreas is exocrine gland-secreting pancreatic fluid into the duodenum after we eat. Throughout the pancreas are tiny clusters of endocrine tissue.

Beta cells that secrete insulin and amylin made of amino acids. Amylin inhibits the secretion of glucagon, slows the emptying of the stomach and sends the "I'm satiated" message to the brain. They reduce the level of glucose in the blood. My Dad stated, "Garbage cans get full, people have a copious abundancy."

Alpha cells secrete glucagon in the liver converting to glucose and fat and protein into intermediate metabolites that also convert to glucose. Both go to the blood to maintain stable blood sugar levels between meals.

Delta cells that secrete somatostatin, which slows down the rate food, are absorbed in the intestine.

Gamma cells secrete pancreatic polypeptide to reduce appetite.

Do not use artificial sweeteners! No snacking between breakfast and lunch. See the chapter on insulin resistance. Movement throughout the day is essential: bike, walk, yoga, treadmill or elliptical, or run up and down a stairway twenty to thirty minutes daily. Take three ten-minute fast walks. Thanks again to Paul Bergner for sharing his CD class on Insulin Resistance.

Visual indications for the pancreas

- Spacey expression, drifting.
- Wet eyes.
- Pasty, gray face.
- Sweating.
- Trembling, shakiness between meals.
- Coated tongue (hyperglycemia).
- Abdominal bloating.
- Abdominal fat (hyperglycemia).
- Underweight (hyperglycemia).
- Overweight (hyperglycemia).
- Edema in feet and legs.
- Pitted nails.
- Slow wound healing (hyperglycemia).

Other indications for the pancreas

- Fatigue (hyperglycemia).
- Gestational diabetes.
- Family history of diabetes (Darn!).
- Frequent peeing (hyperglycemia).
- Dizziness.
- Craving for sweets (hyperglycemia).
- Thirst (hyperglycemia).
- Plenty of saliva.
- High blood pressure.
- Low libido.
- Numbness and tingling of lips.
- Nerve pain in hands and feet (hyperglycemia).
- Burning bottoms of feet.
- Tightened tendon at the bottom of the foot, cramping and needing to stretch it out. Tendon of flexor digitorum longus.
- Weakness in legs.
- Itchy ankles (calcification or red blood cell death), legs, skin especially when going to bed.
- Body pains.
- Constipation.
- Sleepiness after meals.
- Mental disturbances when sugar is out of balance.
- Insomnia: Wake at 3:00 to 4:00 am when adrenals turn on, get up to pee. Eat a little fatty protein in the middle of the night.
- Irritability, snappy.
- Aggressive behavior, or passive aggressive.
- Painful eyes, shooting pain in eyeballs.
- Changes in vision, poor focus relating to liver/glucagon.
- Hunger, instant and immediate "Feed me NOW" (hyperglycemia).
- Weight loss (hyperglycemia).
- Intermittent sweating.

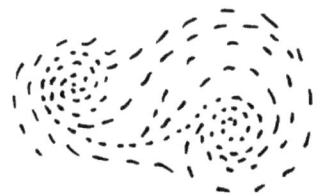

Nutrition for the pancreas

- Breakfast and lunch, eat a palm-sized portion of high protein Omega 3s, grass-fed meats or eggs for breakfast and lunch, with one wholegrain/high fiber all-Pumpernickel or all-Rye toast with olive oil, and dark leafy greens and unheated Cinnamon. Some of the all-Rye breads have Sunflower seeds—great. No snacking between breakfast and lunch.
- Fruits daily 3–4 whole, including ½ cup Blueberries. All berries are beneficial.
- Abundant vegetables, especially Sweet Potatoes, greens, green, orange and yellow vegetables, sprouts.
- Fish (not farm raised).
- Nuts and seeds—soaked overnight in the fridge is best.
- *Al dente* pasta (a little hard).
- 1 apple daily with Sunflower, Peanut or Almond butter.
- Body temperature or warmer water all day.
- A light dinner, salad with a boiled egg, seeds and a few nuts, Sesame dressing or soup.

Avoid or moderate consumption of:

- Juices.
- Alcohol two to four glasses a week (not while pregnant).
- White Potatoes.
- Candy, cake.
- Rare sweets.
- Fried foods, fried chips.
- Refined flour products like bagels, breads, deserts, crackers.

Herbs for the pancreas

- Burdock root.
- Blueberry leaf and Blueberries.
- Chickweed leaf and flower.
- Milk Thistle seed.
- Dandelion root.
- Black Walnut inner hull.
- Licorice root is specific to SI. LI helps cleanse the SI where we make all our coenzymes.

- Green bean juice.
- Gentian root.
- Ginseng root.
- Juniper berry.
- Maitake plus other medicinal mushrooms daily.
- Blue–green algae (not while pregnant unless previously in diet).
- *Pancrease formula*. The late Victoria Fortner of Shawnee Moon Herbaceuticals sent me this formula (1 dropper 2–3 times daily):

• Bitter Melon	• Buchu	• Gymnemma
• Fenugreek	• Garlic	• Pau D'Arco
• Bilberry	• Nettle	• Eleuthero
• Dandelion	• Periwinkle	• Schizandra
• Onion skins	• Red Clover	• Kelp
• Gotu Kola	• Devil's Club	• Ashwaganda

- Plus, John Reddin's Three Ginsengs tonic. (I can formulate for pregnancy.)
- Australian Bush Essence Peach Flowered Tea Tree. 7 drops 2 times daily.
- 3rd Chakra Woodland Essence Flower Essence "digestion and assimilation of experiences." 4 drops twice daily.

Supplements for the pancreas

Supplements **3–4 times daily** with food for three months:

- Chromium 200 mcg.
- EPA-DHA Fish Oil.
- Magnesium glycinate 200 mg.
- Digestive enzymes 2 with meals.
- D3 1,000 IU.

Once daily:

- Zinc liver chelate.
- Vitamin E Wheatgerm oil.
- Q10 Ubiquinol 100 mg.
- B vitamin with intrinsic factor Vessel Care by Metagenics, or sublingual B.

106 AN INTRODUCTION TO *THE PRACTICING HERBALIST*

Twice daily:

- L-carnitine.
- Nightly Triphala (not while pregnant) with 200 Magnesium.
- Multi-mineral.
- Less Vitamin C.

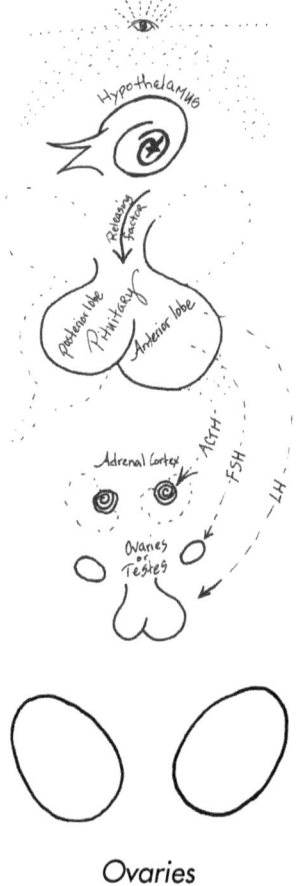

Ovaries

Yes, women are remarkable. A woman has the ability to bleed without dying. Plus we have a lovely receiving room for sperm, warm and moist just right for fertilization and implantation. We can receive sperm from a man or otherwise and become pregnant. On top of that we nourish the fetus during pregnancy, during birthing, and well after the little ones are born and forever more. We are capable of reproducing successfully well into our latter years. My mother carried my daughter's egg in her ovary. Amazing.

Oogenesis is the production of eggs in the ovaries. The ripening follicle of cells surrounding the egg is an endocrine gland making the steroid hormone estrogen for reproductive function and for minimizing loss of calcium from bone (HPA Axis and parathyroid), and promoting blood clotting. Ample estrogen is heart and muscle protective. Estrogen lowers cholesterol and increases libido.

Follicle simulating hormone (FSH) and luteinizing hormone (LH) are inhibited from release by estrogens in the blood except during pre-ovulation when there is an LH SURGE, with a corresponding desire to have sex! Nature, I just love her. Testosterone is needed to have a sex drive. Yes it is.

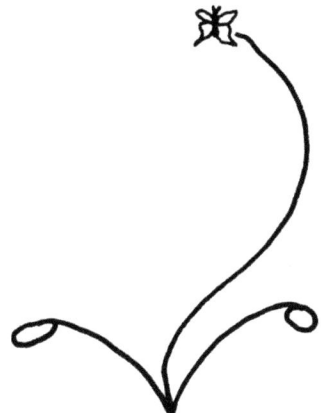

LH from the anterior pituitary binds to receptors that stimulate production of estradiol from cholesterol, which then stimulates the release of the egg. The egg is released; the follicles form a corpus luteum that secretes progesterone.

Progesterone is secreted by the corpus luteum ("yellow body," just like an egg). Progesterone prepares the womb for the baby, halts contractions and another follicle from developing. Progesterone encourages breasts and bones to grow, a healthy womb lining, lowers sensitivity to oxytocin, and is a precursor to androgen and sex hormones. Progesterone helps to maintain Coenzyme Q10 that is essential for heart health.

Estriol-DHEA is weakest and most protective is at the highest level when produced by the placenta.

Women create estradiol metabolites, which are secreted in urine. Esterone is made by muscles and fat. Too much may indicate breast cancer. The last is Estriol.

Estrogen increases when more calories are consumed. Is that where fat and happy came from? All estrogens are metabolized by the liver, secreted in bile or reabsorbed back into the body. Keep that liver healthy!

Visual indications for the ovaries

- Pimple outbreak above or below the lips during ovulation.
- Red, rough, and raised ovarian point above or below lips (high estrogen).
- Vertical lines above the lips. Cessation of ovarian function on that side.
- Wide hips.
- Abundant breasts.
- Hair growth around genitals and armpits.
- Adipose (fat) tissue contributing to a shapely appearance.
- Non-healing cystic acne.
- Pale and bleeding gums (lack of progesterone to make Coenzyme Q10 ubiquinol).
- Voluptuous breasts and buttocks (estrogen excess).
- Wrist looks gray from blood stagnation (Angelica). M.W.

Other indications for the ovaries

- Infertility. Look to history of sexually transmitted diseases: Chlamydia, gonorrhea, etc. or the formation of scar tissue from endometriosis or intrinsic factor deficiency.
- Muscle pain.
- Extreme pain during menstrual cycle.
- History of sexual abuse.
- Edema, water weight increased in hands, feet, cranium prior to period (progesterone excess).
- Increased appetite prior to period (progesterone excess).
- Neurotic behavior prior to period (progesterone excess): "I want to ... somebody."
- Rx of progesterone get a bad response.
- Miscarriages (use Solomon's Seal, Black Haw, Raspberry, Wild Yam, Vitex and Partridge berry) (progesterone deficiency).

- High blood sugar (progesterone excess).
- "Excess estrogen: short periods, bright blood, tender breasts the week prior to bleeding, hot body temp, pain at ovulation. Voluptuous breasts and buttocks, fibroids in endometrium, endometriosis, wrist looks gray from blood stagnation (Angelica)." M.W.

Nutrition for the ovaries

- Eggs.
- Seeds.
- Foods that reproduce.

Herbs for the ovaries

Three- and six-leaved plants support the reproductive organs.

- Black Cohosh root.
- White Peony root is good for liver-processing hormones and liver wind.
- Milky Oats aerial parts.
- Chickweed leaf and flower.
- Blessed Thistle aerial parts.
- Cramp Bark.
- Alfalfa aerial parts.
- Blue Vervain aerial parts (progesterone excess). Too intense above, weakened below, neurotic, stiff. M.W.
- Shepherd's Purse aerial parts (progesterone excess), weak expulsive powers, clots and cramps, fibroids in muscles, dropped uterus. "Ambitious women." M.W.
- False Unicorn root (endangered, plant a few and nurture, gather one and tincture).
- Yarrow aerial parts. Yarrow is progesterone antagonist—controls excess bleeding.
- Trillium root: "Uterus flooded with blood, expulsive, endometriosis, excess bleeding after delivery, collapse of pelvic contents and tenderness." M.W.
- She Oak. Australian Bush Essence. 7 drops twice daily.
- Ovaries 2nd and 3rd chakras, creativity, self, relationships, emotions, sensuality.

Supplements for the ovaries

- Evening Primrose Oil.
- Vitamin E Wheatgerm oil.

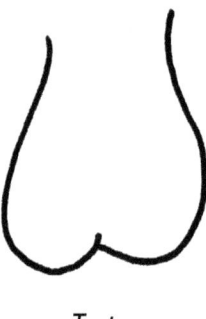

Testes

The testes produce sperm (100 million a day) for reproductive function. Testes also produce testosterone for development of sex characteristics: deep voice, body and beard hair, and a manly shape. Wear loosely fitting underwear: "swingies not clingies" for sperm development.

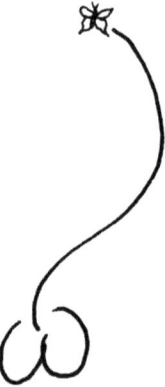

Luteinizing Hormone acts on interstitial cells (Leydig cells) of the testes, stimulating them to synthesize and secrete testosterone. Interstitial cell stimulating hormone (ICSH) in men is simply LH. All is under the control of from the pituitary and hypothalamus. Testosterone is needed to produce sperm. DHT is a form of testosterone that has greater stability in some target tissues. Inhibin is for inhibiting FSH via action on the pituitary. Progesterone and testosterone both compete for the same receptor sites. The DHEA (same as cortisol) pathway can be produced by testes and adrenals.

Nature is so powerful! When my Mom was diagnosed with leukemia, and told she had months to live, my Dad suddenly was able to have erections again. As death approached his primal instincts kicked his endocrine system into action for the survival of the species.

Visual indications for the testes

- Abnormal genital development (LH receptor) (mutations in the genes encoding the androgen receptor).
- Effeminate features (GnRH receptor) (mutations in the genes encoding the androgen receptor) (low testosterone).
- Blocked development of gonads in males and females (FSH receptor) (mutations in the genes encoding the androgen receptor).
- Large breasts (low testosterone): look to excessive Cannabis consumption.
- Abundant body fat (low testosterone).
- Losing scalp hair (high testosterone).
- Very muscular (high testosterone).
- Persistent erection (high testosterone). Hopefully not seen in consultation but heard about.

Other indications for the testes

- Abnormal sexual function in males (mutations of encoded genes).
- High-pitched voice.
- Lean body (high testosterone).
- Redness, dryness above and below lips.
- Carbohydrate craving (low testosterone).
- Infertility, low sperm count (low testosterone).
- Aggressive behavior (high testosterone).
- Loves to eat meat (high testosterone).
- Bloating.
- Low libido (low testosterone).

Nutrition for the testes

- Bowls of seeds and nuts, Pumpkin especially.
- Oysters (Doctrine of signatures).
- Figs (more Doctrine of signatures).

Herbs for the testes

- Sassafras root. "My understanding of this via Matthew and Stephen Buhner is different—what I learned is that Sarsaparilla does two things to normalize testosterone—provides steroidal precursors and aids in liver clearance of testosterone to allow the hypothalamus to get a fresh read on testosterone levels in the bloodstream and reset accordingly, thus increasing or decreasing it as needed. Pine Pollen definitely is straight usable testosterone, though," shares Sean Donahue.
- Scots Pine Pollen.
- Burdock root.
- American Ginseng root.
- Sarsaparilla root "straight usable plant testosterone." P.D.L.
- Saw Palmetto berry—take with fat.
- Wild Yam root.
- Damiana aerial parts.
- Angelica root.
- Black Cohosh root.

CHAPTER 6

Examining color

The following tables list colors in various parts of the body with opinions concerning possible health issues to look for. These are the combined teachings of Matthew Wood and David Winston and their teacher William LeSassier. "Always look to three areas for confirmation," reminds David Winston.

White

"There are several different kinds of white. It can indicate deficiency from lack of blood or circulation, tension squeezing out the blood, or cold from lack of circulation." M.W. Look to pale nail beds and sclera. Leaky kidney—low back pain, knee pain, excess peeing.

The following table summarizes indications associated with the color white:

Indicator		Association
TONGUE	White patches on edge	Possible sign of cancer. Refer to a medical doctor. AIDS
	White frothy "runners" down sides between stomach area and the edge	Spleen damp and cold or lymphatic system damp and cold
	White coating	Cold, yeast, candida, mucus, dampness into phlegm
	White dots	Scarlet fever, deep cold
CHEEKS	White blotches (leukoplakia)	Dental issues. AIDS. Syphilis
STOOLS	White, greasy stools	May be celiac disease, a gluten allergy
	White, dry stools	Lack of bile, gallbladder weakness, poor small intestine assimilation
	Mucus in stool	Stomach or large intestine secreting mucus (if nauseated). Colitis
NAILS	Pale when pressed	Anemia
EYEBALL	Ring around	Intense pain, anemia
LOWER LID	Pull down and pale	Anemia

Green

The following table summarizes indications associated with the color green:

Indicator	Association
HAIR	Aluminum poisoning
HAIR and FINGERNAIL BEDS, infertility	Copper toxicity, Shákoon
FECES	High consumption of chlorophyll or artificial grape coloring
SKIN	Hyperparathyroid. P.D.L.

Other indicators for aluminum poisoning include anger, diarrhea, nausea, skin rashes, arthritis, and memory loss.

Red

In general, deep pink nails and gums, and a pink overall skin tone indicate health. This implies good blood circulation. A healthy tongue is a lovely pink to red. Angry red coloration; yes, the liver grows to adapt, creates more veins, and is less simple. We do live in the "United Inebriated Nations," joked William LeSassier.

The following table summarizes indications associated with the color red:

Indicator		Association
Excess red (anywhere), carmine, pink/red indicates a higher activity of heat. M.W. Dark red indicates a lower, smoldering heat. M.W.		Heat in the system, inflammation, high blood pressure, or heart issue
FACE	Red	A robust, sanguine person, full of blood. Tends to willfulness, injuries, enthusiasm, and over-exertion. Needs a sedative. M.W.
TONGUE TIP	Red	Disturbed heart, insomnia, manic behavior With coat—drain Without coat—supplement. M.W.
SKIN	Red skin rashes	Heat. Blood disorders, allergies, autoimmune diseases, arthritis, lupus, drug reactions, rosacea or infections
	Red dots	Heat, too much sugar in the system causing heat
PALMS	Red palms and skin tissues that when you press on them take a long time for white to return to red	Oxygenation, heat. Hawthorn. M.W.
	Red mole-like dots	Heat in the system. (Lalou Bégué)

(Continued)

(Continued)

Indicator		Association
CHEEK	One red, one cheek pale	Heat and tension. Fever. (Chamomile)
	Dusky, darkish red	Septic heat. Needs a stimulant
	"Clown cheeks"; red capillaries	Redness from fever
	Rosy red circles after meals	Babies—food allergy
NOSE	Red nose	Heart condition, rosacea or alcoholism
	Red tip of nose	Heart issues
	Red nostril edges	Stomach irritation
	Big, bulbous nose	A heart problem
	Broken blood vessels on nose	Alcohol abuse, lack of bioflavonoids
	Red bridge of nose	Infection burning down into tissues. Upper respiratory/lungs. Cartilaginous tissue
	Red extending down from nostrils	Heat, oxygenation. Hawthorn. M.W.
EARS	Red upper outer edge of ears	Liver fire rising, headaches, high blood pressure
	Whole ear red	Earaches, high blood pressure
EYES	Red conjunctiva of eye	Allergies, contacts, chlorine, foreign particles. "Have eaten a food with spices or red coloring?"
	Red conjunctiva of eye, itchy, hot, mucusy, like glass is in the eye	Conjunctivitis—contagious.
	Red outer corner of eye	Spleen. W.Le.
	Bump on lid	Stye, blepharitis, ingrown eyelash. Hot compress of: Calendula, Plantain, Elder Flower, Goldenseal, or Red Clover

(Continued)

(Continued)

Indicator		Association
EYES SOCKET	Orange coloration on inside of socket	Long-term lack of assimilation of Vitamin A, leukemia
	Red puffy outer eye socket	Food allergy
SCLERA	Red sclera between pupil and nose	Colon, liver or stomach inflammation, constipation
TONGUE	Papillae	Lymph and immune systems
	Raised red papillae	A systemic infection. Looks like little red dots. Often been on antibiotics. Low-grade infection Old infections
	Pink/red or carmine, dark red	Excess heat, autoimmune, excess blood to surface capillaries—need for sedatives. Melissa, Peach, Rose, Hawthorn, Wild Cherry, and Yarrow. M.W.
	Dark red	Deep infection, chronic. (Dandelion)
	Magenta, carmine	Extreme heat, B-2/riboflavin deficiency, blood stasis, thrombosis. (Yarrow). M.W.
	Red/orange	Pernicious anemia (B-12 shots)
	Purple; dark, dark red	Low-grade septic infection or rashes where toxic materials are coming to the surface. Heart or lung disease. Echinacea, Phytolacca
	Red tongue tip	Mind, heart, lungs overactive—use sedatives
	Red center tongue	Stomach, digestive system
	Red lower tongue	Intestine, kidneys, reproductive system
GUMS	Red, swollen, bleeding	Gingivitis (poor dental hygiene, oral sex), anemia, leukemia, Vitamin C deficiency

Gray

The following table summarizes indications associated with the color gray: Gray coloration indicates a lack of oxygenation and depletion.

Indicator		Association
FACE	Ashen gray	Lung, shock, dehydration, too much carbon monoxide
	Yellow/gray complexion with blue/purple tones around veins	Poor lipid metabolism (Angelica). M.W.
CHEEKS	Hollow and gray	Depressed lung function, tobacco, emphysema, and marijuana. Pimples, psoriasis, may not be eliminating wastes through lungs. Deep breathing is paramount. "Gray coloration in the cheeks indicates poor oxidation from the lungs or tight capillaries. Tension." M.W.
SCLERA	Gray sclera	Constipation or sluggish bowels
TONGUE	Gray mucus on back third	Sluggish bowel, constipation, smoking, and excess heat. Smoking creates little holes in the roof of your mouth. Gross
	Dirty, gray coloring	Looks just like *Echinacea angustifolia* root. Use it. Also Red Root

Yellow

Yellow is associated with stagnation of digestion and assimilation in the stomach, spleen, lymphatics, liver, and gallbladder.

The following table summarizes indications associated with the color yellow:

Indicator	Association
Yellow around mouth and nose	Stagnant digestion
Yellow around eyes with bumps	Fatty deposits. Look to liver/ gallbladder
Yellow around mouth, nose and eyes, with red cheeks	A specific indication for Yellow Dock. M.W.
Sallow complexion	Digestion/assimilation/weakness
General yellowness	Hepatitis, jaundice (eyes first, hands, then skin), obstruction of bile
Yellow tongue coating	Same as white but with heat
Yellow skin	Hypervitaminosis A
Yellow skin and whites of eyes	Jaundice

Orange

Indicator	Association
Inner orbit of eye socket	Lack of assimilation of carotenoids. Leukemia

Blue

Blue indicates lack of oxygen, stagnant venous blood, and dehydration. Low blood pressure, can't handle cold, joints may be stiff.

The following table summarizes indications associated with the color blue:

Indicator		Association
TONGUE	Blue tongue body	Can be poor circulation, heart disease, impaired respiration, asthma, or internal dampness
	Blue tongue body	Before the period the tongue will be blue
	Blue tongue body, menopausal	"Give remedies and the period will come." M.W.
	Red tongue with blue center, flame-shaped	Specific indication for Yarrow. M.W.

(Continued)

(Continued)

Indicator		Association
MOUTH	Bluish white spots surrounded by red	Measles
EYE	Sclera is clear/bluish	Poor circulation or anemia
	Whites of eyes are blue	Lack of circulation
Below Eye	Blue–black "allergic shiners" under the eye, like a black eye	Food allergies or other long-term allergies; low immunity; marrow and kidneys decreased
	Blue–black pencil line under eye on orbital ridge	Always a specific food allergy, like chocolate
Beside Eye	Light blue, puffy, outer corner going toward cheek	Intense pain

Black

The following table summarizes indications associated with the color black:

Indicator		Association
SKIN	Pitch black bruises	Stagnant blood. Very old people. Encourage massage and use fresh Yarrow tincture or oil
	Black, sooty complexion	Blood stagnation, specific for Sassafras. M.W.
	Black complexion, dark circles within orbit of eye	Normal appearance for Mediterranean, East Indian, African heritage
	Blue–black pencil line under eyes at top of cheek bone	Chronic food allergies. Adrenal corticol exhaustion
	Blue–black like a bruise under the eyes	Liver stagnation with food allergies, too much fried food, environmental allergies

(*Continued*)

(Continued)

Indicator		Association
	Blue–black translucent band under the eyes with pale skin	Constitutional weak immunity, low nutrition, lack of sleep, low bone marrow function (low immunity, red blood cells, low kidney function). Adrenal deficiency: try Eleuthero or Spikenard. W.Le.
TONGUE	Blue–black tongue sides	Liver. Fringe Tree bark, says Christopher Hobbs
	Black on tongue	Often seen on very old people's tongues
	Blue–black tongue, middle	Digestion
	Black mark on tongue	Stagnant blood in the spine, uterus or elsewhere. Use Knotweed with a black mark on it. M.W.
VEINS	Blue–black, swollen, surrounded by yellow	Stagnant and putrid blood. (White Oak bark)

"Dark circles under the eyes, give Siberian Ginseng (now named Siberian Eleuthero) and watch the circles go, said William LeSassier. Indicates adrenal exhaustion. William also gave Spikenard—more for women," quotes Matthew Wood.

Purple

VEINS	Blue–black, swollen veins that look like grapes	White Oak bark tincture, 3 drops, 1–3 times daily. Caused by a lack of tone in veins. Runners who sit the rest of the day
TONGUE	Purple and stiff	Extreme stagnant blood in the heart
LIPS	Purple	Extreme stagnant blood in the heart
FINGER-NAILS	Purple at cuticle and tip White center	Extreme lack of circulation

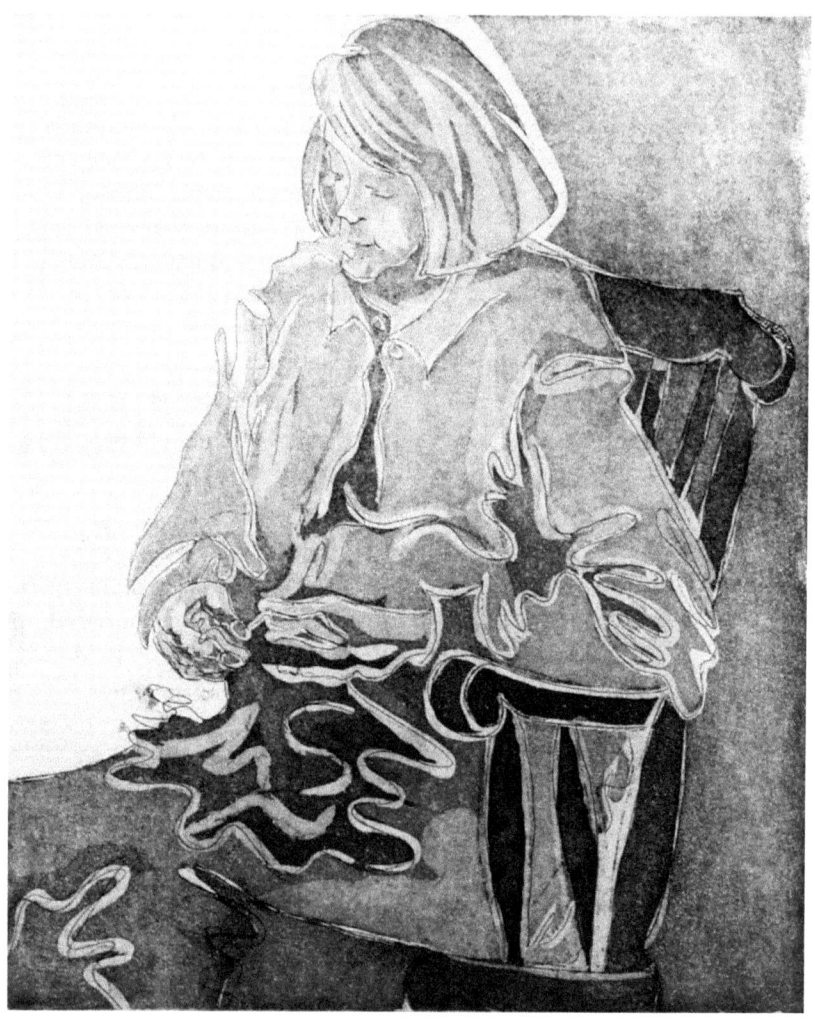

Kaiya in the Rocker

CHAPTER 7

Organ/body correspondences

Emotional and physical reflexes are signals that are sent to one area of the body to let you know there is a problem in another part of the body.
They should get a medical diagnosis, but even then, they may want a more "organic" and "profound" or "insightful" look at what is going on in the organs. Matthew Wood

Stomach

The stomach corresponds to the nose and upper lip and the toe next to the big toe. Digestive problems are indicated by rashes or pimples near the edge of the nostrils. *Gut instincts. Courage.*

The stomach also reflexes to the tongue in general. The surface of the tongue reveals the absolute condition of your interior. The central area of the tongue is the stomach. A lot of crevices indicate poor digestion. Many people are born with a dividing line, so a dividing line is not necessarily diagnostic. The central line is the line of digestion in general; it is also the line of the spine. If you have a wiggle in your central line, you may have scoliosis, a cervical problem, or something turned or bulging in the spine. The front part of the tongue corresponds to the cervical spine.

If you have crevices in the tongue that are irritated and going off to the side, the more red and irritated-looking they are, the more heat is in the system. This may be indigestion, too much hydrochloric acid, or gastric ulcer, or lack of intrinsic factor. Excess acids will show up as a vertical, central deep line on the bottom lip and sometimes the top lip. This line may indicate an ulcer when red in the center. Hanging skin from the back of arms indicates low stomach acid. The pituitary gland is related to stomach issues.

Gum problems and mouth ulcers indicate stomach heat. M.W. Fermentation of foods is indicated by gas—upper or lower. Bloating can occur from stagnation in the stomach caused by too little stomach fire or too many fluids while eating meals. Amylase is required for good digestion. Avoid toothpaste with glycerin in it! Try making your own!

The upper lip, if it is pale, means there is not enough digestive fire going to the stomach and not enough blood circulating through the system. Paleness is always a lack of blood. M.W.

Keeping the mouth open all the time indicates blocked sinus or poor digestion. Lines on the right side of the lips going down to the corner of the chin refer to the duodenum (look to the pancreas and bile flow). Mouth sores, red dot in white circle, indicate excess heat (needs vitamin E).

The pyloric valve reflexes to the left corner of the mouth going down to meet the chin. Look at the corner of your mouth and draw a line down and across following the dent above your chin; that is the area of the pyloric valve. People with pylorus issues have a lot of deep, irritated-looking lines coming down from their mouths. They're not producing enough enzymes so they're not digesting their foods enough. These cracks in particular can be vitamin B deficiencies. B vitamins are the first to go under stress. Elders don't die of old age; they die of starvation. They're eating foods but not receiving benefits from them. If there is redness and irritation there is heat.

Small intestine

The small intestine reflexes to the lower half of the forehead. Choppy short lines there indicate inner stress. The feeling of being tired 1½ hours after eating indicates small intestine, as well as being tired daily between

1:00 and 3:00 pm. The emotion of being overwhelmed is another indication. Enthusiasm or lack of it. The small intestine relates to the effective intake of nutrition. How you take in your world. For elders and others who are thin and emaciated, look to lack of assimilation.

The digestive process simply stated is all started in the mouth—saliva, good stomach digestion—proper acid balance, and good pancreas and bile function—small intestine assimilation. Look to the lines connecting the chin to the outer corner of the lips, which indicates small intestine spasticity. Narrow feces may indicate Crohn's, irritable bowel, colitis, or a fibroid pressing on the intestine. Well, perhaps it begins with the hand bringing the spoon to the mouth.

Frontal headaches point to the small intestine, as do small red pimples with scaling (leaky gut). All rashes on the lower forehead point to poor reaction of food in the small intestine. The small intestine is another "worry organ."

Large intestine

The large intestine reflexes to the upper forehead, fingernails, and the area between the cheek and nose. This area starts from the upper area beside the nose and heads downward to the outer corners of the lips. Large intestine lines are some of the easiest to read and some of the most dramatic. The depth, pouching, forking, and shapes running along this line are all indicators of the tone, transit time, and vitality of the organ. You can envision fecal matter, building up in the alimentary canal and pouching over. If the bottom of the large intestine line forks and has an inverted "V" closing it to create a diamond-shaped island, that may indicate a tumor that is growing and impairing normal flow. Stagnation. You can see pouching with people who eat too much brown rice, too much meat, too much dense food. Bread lovers. They need fiber. You know: fruit, lots of veggies, salads, and exercise.

Another large intestine area to note is the upper forehead. The horizontal lines, their length and number, indicate the state of the nervous system connected to the large intestine. Blueness within lines on the forehead or cheek is a lack of oxygen going to the large intestine—so a lack of blood as well.

As Matthew Wood says, the purpose of the large intestine is "to make a nice stool, a little last stop digestion." In America we live in the land of "holding on," constipation. The large intestine is all about holding on to old, hmmm, stuff. In order to make a nice stool, we need balance in the intake of water, fiber, and nutrient-rich foods, as well as daily physical movement, fresh air, and a forgiving attitude. Supplementing with bioflora (including acidophilus, bifidus, and *Streptococcus thermophilus*) plus soaked Chia or Flax seeds, eating yogurt or kefir and taking mucilaginous herbs like Slippery Elm and Marshmallow, helps maintain a healthy intestine. A perfect bowel movement is brown, perfectly formed, gently released, gracefully curling into the toilet bowl without splashing, and no visible food parts. "Colonvana," as Matt defines them.

Some symptoms of large intestine problems include headache at the base of the skull and tension in the muscles. People who get muscle tension and then get a headache. I'll poke away at their shoulders and feel the hardness of the tissue, see what the resistance is, check if the muscle hardness extends along the trapezius muscle—which holds that heavy head up. Irritable bowel, diverticulosis, diverticulitis, colitis, and constipation, all indicate stress and inflammation instead of good peristalsis. Skin rashes and breakouts, and candida, indicate "leaky gut" instead of healthy tight pores in the walls of intestinal mucosa.

The large intestine is all about feeling safe and the ability to let go.

Liver

The liver reflexes to the eyes. Any change in vision—focus being dull, then improving later in the day; thickening of the tissues (cataracts); wet or dry eye—all reflex to the liver. The liver also reflexes to the big toe, near the outer edges of the inner nail bed. The emotional expression is anger expressed or anger held in. "The smooth flow of emotions across the body," as William LeSassier said. Have you ever noticed how alcoholics rage? All that firewater is hard on the liver. Raging alcoholic. Alcohol abuse is just looking for God, or the god within, in the wrong direction. Eighty-five percent of our population is either directly in relationship with an alcoholic, or one indirectly affects their lives. The liver is the metabolic headquarters for the body.

"Fire and fuel (blue blood) and air (red blood) and valve (autonomic nervous system) equals smooth metabolic flow. Otherwise, toxins build up, creating issues like allergies, blood sugar conditions, cholesterol imbalances and hormonal issues. Malnutrition also becomes an issue indicated by heat, dry or congestion (damp)." M.W.

Some indications include a central vertical line between the eyes. Sighing constantly is a sign of liver Chi stagnation—life is too much for you. The ears tone a low droning sound; there may be headaches at the temporal lobe. Clear floaters in the line of vision indicate anemia; dark floaters indicate toxicity. Worrying about the future. The pointer (index) finger reflexes to the liver.

Gallbladder

The gallbladder reflexes to the temple and is indicated by tics and twitches. The headache is "an icepick in the temple." It also reflexes to the toe next to the little toe. Lack of "egoic will" manifests in gallbladder issues. Passive aggressive behavior. Feeling galled. Well, she had a lot of gall! The gallbladder manages bile. When out of balance, you can't eat fats and process them. "A little job, big importance." M.W.

People always have indigestion with gallbladder issues, and after a high fat meal they feel pain or discomfort in the gallbladder and liver area. Pain can refer into the back and over the shoulders and be excruciating! Bloating, tics, and clay stools are other symptoms. A gallbladder headache comes over the left right side, up from the back and over the front. Right temple headache. Gallbladder people often have prominent blue veins on the sides of their faces. The angrier they get, the more the veins stick out. Veins sticking out can also be a heart issue. Heart-related issues are often red veins, and the gallbladder ones are more blue.

William always said, "Pay attention to where you're itching." If you have an itch, what organ is it over? That's very interesting to me. So if you have an itch somewhere constantly, go to your anatomy book and see what organ is underneath there. Good advice.

The coloration of a gallbladder circle under the eye is brown to yellow, all gradations of yellow to brown. Dandruff is a sign of gallbladder issue. There's a difference between dandruff and dry scalp. Dandruff sticks to the hair; dry scalp doesn't. People who produce a lot of earwax will often have a gallbladder issue—interesting. Often the wax buildup is in one ear. Wax is kind of sticky and oily. Look for yellow colorations in sclera, skin, and tongue coating.

People with gallbladder problems also often have boundary issues. They either have no boundaries, walking into a home unannounced, or into private body parts inappropriately, or live alone away from everyone. When I interview a client, I always try to mix up the emotional components, the societal components, the physical symptoms, because you'll get as much in a conversation with a person about how they're living as what you're seeing from the lines.

> *You need good boundaries to be open*
> *Healthy boundaries allow our hearts to be fully Open*
>
> — KARYN SANDERS

Spleen/pancreas

From 9:00 to 11:00 am you worry about work. The spleen produces white blood cells and stores excess red cells. It is an integral part of the immune system. The spleen is another worry organ. People who think too much have a spleen issue—the entire Vata population of the world. Spleen issues show up as prolapses of any kind: prolapsed uterus, prolapsed rectum, prolapsed bladder, prolapsed intestine. Men have as many of these issues as women, except that men have prostate issues. It is all about thinking. You know, I think all the time. The hardest thing for me to do is shut it off. So what do I have to do? Meditate.

"The spleen is like the scrap heap of the blood system because it removes broken down red-blood cells from the blood and rejuvenates the good ones for further use," John Courtney said. Very ecological.

One indication will be little choppy lines across the forehead. Also on the face, these lines come down the side of the face from the outer edge of the eye and wash down into the cheek. Think of a rainfall in the desert, or being at the beach when the waves recede. You will see little rivulets, lines that wiggle down. They look like those dried rivulets at the ocean's edge. Those are spleen lines. They're different from laugh lines. When anyone scrunches their face, they have those little 'crow's feet.' Those lines are just laugh lines or being out in the sun too much. To check that, ask somebody, "Are you a landscaper? Are you out in the sun all the time?" They will have facial lines just from working outdoors. Weathered—what does the sun do? It melts the protective fat layer in your skin. The skin becomes leathery. The cheek may be sunken, which may indicate wasting of the spleen or lung. Doug Simons recommends Chaparral oil for "all conditions of the sun." Coconut oil is also wonderful.

People who bloat and swell after eating have congestion in the stomach and spleen. Taking astringents prior to meals and taking in less water will help. W.Le. Look to intrinsic factor deficiency.

People who dwell on the past are spleen people. For example, somebody got divorced but twenty years later they're still really angry. Still dwelling on the money, time, and hopes lost. Whatever.

People with spleen issues have a tendency to get styes in their eyes. They tend to have redness in the outer corners of their eyes. The most common injury to the spleen is dampness. So a lot of New Englanders, where I'm from, have spleen issues.

Look for pain on the left side under the ribs, low appetite, sallow to yellow skin, scanty urine, and weakness.

Pale lips indicate not enough blood in the stomach and spleen. The stomach energy consumes all their blood, or, they don't have enough heat and blood produced. This is what William LeSassier calls "stomach anemia." Absence of fire. Eat warming foods between 7:00 and 9:00 am.

Another indication is scalloped edges on the tongue. It takes a tremendous amount of pressure from inner tension to make these indentations. People with puffy, scalloped tongues benefit from drinking tea of Poria. Lalou Bégué, my acupuncturist for twenty years, and William both have suggested this white curly shaving of fungus. "Poria dries and astringes the abdominal." Also try Goldenrod, *Solidago canadensis* tea—the leaves—as an infusion.

"Cook Slippery Elm, cut and sifted (one tight handful to 32 ounces cold water), and decoct until it has separated. The color is blood red and the texture is about that of blood. At that point, though it still has an action on the colon, I think its primary action is on the spleen. Love and Light." P.D.L.

Without a spleen there is more risk of infection. Be cautious with fevers. Thomas Bartram suggests using New Jersey tea (Red Root). My experience with Red Root is that it opens blocked or severed channels to allow an even flow.

When there are spleen issues, a white, tiny kidney bean shape pops out along the inner eye socket. I have had clients who were in high-speed car accidents. Bang, the sudden stop, and the organs fly forward. And all of a sudden, this little kidney bean pops out above the eye. It can appear on either eye socket. Even when people have their spleen removed the kidney bean seems to stay forever. With a car accident it can be there and then after a number of years go away. But if the organ is removed, that little kidney bean appears to stay. Diabetics also tend to have the spleen bean.

Enlarged spleen may indicate anemia, leukemia, or malaria. When swollen, the spleen bulges out like a football at the side of the torso along the rib tips. Use Thuja. I haven't seen malaria yet. Herbs to consider besides Red Root are Goldenseal, Bayberry, Echinacea, Barberry, Dandelion, and Fringe Tree bark. Chemotherapy? Try Astragalus; Agrimony when irritable. Add B-12, methylcobalamin sublingually, zinc, vitamin A, and soluble iron to support the spleen.

The pancreas deals with blood sugar and relates to spleen directly.

Lungs

The lungs correspond to the cheeks. Gray coloration indicates toxins or lack of vital energy; white indicates shock. Sunken cheeks indicate wasting of the lung or spleen. Rippling lines may run up the cheeks to the center of the eye socket.

Lungs also correspond to the index finger. The nails flip up when a person has asthma. When nails are spongy and barely attached, TB, bronchitis, cancer, or cystic fibrosis are indicated. A blue line at the cuticle, especially the thumb, indicates a lack of oxygen. Lungs represent all conditions affecting breathing.

Good lung and heart circulation can be read on fingernails. The more moons on fingernails the better. Lunula, luneria, those half-moons at the tips of fingernails.

Lungs hold the emotion of worry and unresolved sorrow. Kapha = damp lung, Vata = dry lung. I had a client with emphysema hold in all of the unexpressed sorrow from her childhood, her son's death, and other frustrations in her life. She didn't allow her tears to fall. She applied the barriers of smoke, make up, and carried the "tough girl" attitude with her. In order to become well, complete her journey, she had to learn how to express sorrow. Nancy Anne Risley taught that the air pathway in Polarity (pointer finger, throat chakra, lungs) is where lung imbalance shows. Shoulders correspond to the lungs. Elbows indicate the triple heater or heart. W.Le. Shallow breathers and asthmatics often have horizontal lines at the bridge of the nose.

"The liver, gallbladder and stomach all feed the lungs. In Chinese medicine the adrenals and thyroid are the gateway to the lung. The pointer finger and thumb, fold the other fingers back and you have a gun." W.Le.

Kidneys

The kidneys reflex to the ears. Kids with ear infections can be eating too many mucus-forming foods. Their eustachian tubes are too little to handle any swelling. Take them off dairy, wheat, and corn. They may also be hearing arguing or too much loudness in the home. The ears will have a high-pitched ring (tinnitus), be itchy and dry, or painful to the touch. Palms of the hands may itch. Puffiness under the eyes indicates kidney imbalance. Great herbs for these water issues are Sweet Leaf (*Monarda fistulosa*) in small-drop doses and Dandelion leaf. Often there is edema. The imprint of socks or wrist marks stay on the body with edema.

Kidneys hold the emotions of fear, lack of will and power. Experiences of sexual abuse are held in the reproductive organs and thighs.

Big earlobes indicate good kidney energy. A diagonal line in the earlobe indicates a collapsed capillary bed, in part from a lack of water. William always said, "Pull on your ears to get a better constitution." Ears are inverted embryos; any tender points indicate pathology. Large ears are strong constitution, strong kidney energy, and long ears indicate longevity. On the time clock 3:00 to 5:00 pm is the kidney doldrums time. W.Le.

When the ear disappears into the head and doesn't have delineation the constitution is weaker. Outside ankles point to bladder. Inside ankles point to kidney.

When working with end-stage cancer clients, use some caution if they have edema. If the fluids are worked upward, they will fill the lungs, bringing on pain and respiratory failure.

Bladder

The bladder reflexes to the pelvic region, inside ankle point, little toe and the hairline. There is also a little puffy blue point on the acupuncture bladder point, on the arch of the foot at the most curved point.

The pelvic region, including the bladder, may store past sexual abuse. Diseases include cystitis, interstitial cystitis and/or dysfunction of the reproductive organs. Symptoms are prolapse of the bladder, pain during urination, pain during intercourse, cystitis after intercourse, breakouts or dandruff at the hairline.

Pelvic floor

The pelvis reflexes to the jaw. Chi, feeling centered. The jaw line mimics the line of the pelvic floor. If you were to lift up the pelvis and superimpose it onto the jaw line, you can read the location. Does a pimple appear at the lower cheek at ovulation each month, alternating sides, or only break out on the odd months? (Ovaries). Is there a breakout around the lips just prior to bleeding? (Uterus). Are there vertical lines above the lips, one side or both? (Lack of ovarian function). Are there pimples along the jaw line? Look to stagnation in the pelvic floor, hip issues, pelvic inflammatory disease.

Brown pigmentation on the jaw indicates pelvic toxicity and a connection to imbalance in the pineal gland.

"Acniform sores on the chin (red, sore, similar to acne), especially at ovulation, equal high estrogen, estrogen stress, or bleeding/cramping (test White Peony root). A constant angry red pimple over the ovary area may be a fibroid or tumor. A small chin indicates less water element (reproductive energy). A large, cleft chin indicates being driven by the reproductive organs." W.Le.

Did the person just get their teeth cleaned a few weeks prior to the onset of pelvic floor problems? The bacteria in the human mouth are strong and when the teeth are cleaned they are dumped directly into the lymphatic system. Sublingual (under the tongue) is the fastest route to the entire bloodstream. Scrape bacteria and plaque off the teeth and off it goes. Systemically. Ask if they have had an abscessed tooth. Take two squirts of Echinacea and Calendula every four hours the day before and after teeth are cleaned.

Heart

The heart corresponds to the shape and coloration of the tongue and nose. High blood pressure shows as red coloration on the curled edges of the ears. Variations in red coloration on the face in general indicate heart issues. Heart is the expression of joy that is under- or over-expressed or given and received. The heart is "the King," as William said. "One never goes directly to the King. All other organs work for the well-being of the King and therefore the kingdom prospers." Pitta relates to the heart. Treat the other organs that feed the heart, drain away from the heart.

Palpitations are often hyperthyroidism or nervousness. A slow beat indicates the Kapha body type and lethargy. M.W. An irregular heartbeat indicates poor electrical connections. Reddish complexion indicates heat in the heart or rosacea. Cold hands and feet indicate poor circulation through the venous system, thyroid imbalance, heart disease, or diabetes.

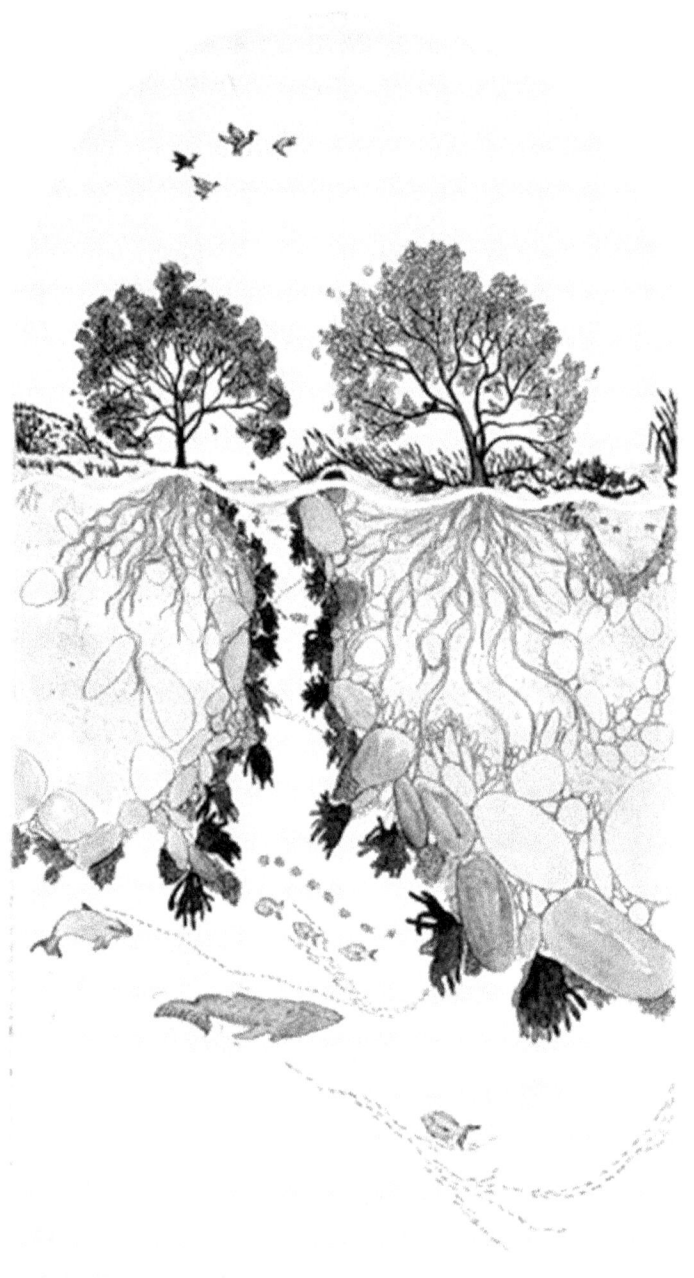

September morning

CHAPTER 8

Await indications of three

Here are some visual signs to look for as your clients sit before you. Remember to use them as references not absolutes. Look to three areas before passing judgment. Mark down your own observations. Remember these words of the late William LeSassier: "The oscillation between certainty and uncertainty—don't look at just one indication."

These first came to me through a special friend and teacher, David Winston, who has shared much great knowledge through the years. He learned from William LeSassier when they were both young men. William became my teacher over twenty years later. I also have studied with Christopher Hobbs and am constantly learning these skills from Matthew Wood. Matt has become my brother bear. We teach together and learn from each other. I am grateful for the depth of wisdom all my teachers offer.

Please remember that I do not know everything. These are indicators I have learned from teachers and from viewing many clients. Everything changes in time. These are tools to use. And just like your garden tools, clean them up, sand them down and refinish them once in a while.

Assess a client visually as well as asking questions and interpreting responses. Have a low-intensity flashlight handy to shine on the client's face. Of course, avoid shining the light directly in the eyes. Try to have good natural light in the room. Ask them to come without nail polish and make-up. They should not eat foods that will color the tongue prior to consultation.

Look to the constitution of the person, the energetics of the condition and the energetics of the herbs. A generality to define a good constitution is that they will have strong, even, well-defined features. The bushier the eyebrows, the fuller the ear lobe, the better the ability to recover from illness and adversity. Share positive indications: they empower the person to call on their inner healing powers.

Our tools: the wisdom of our teachers, our choice of words, use of hands, our thoughts, the objects in our office, a Biomat or AmpCoil in conjunction with herbs are all choices to have in the practitioner's toolbox.

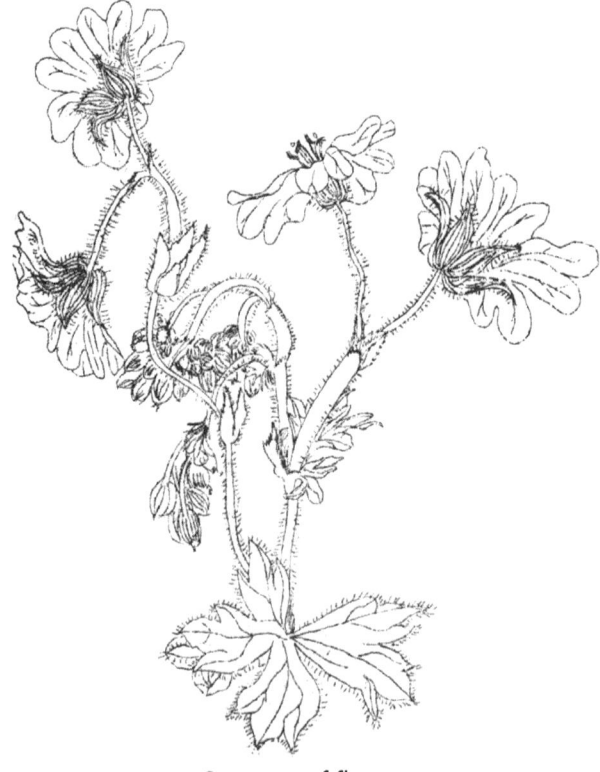

Segment of flower

CHAPTER 9

Examining the face

Be sure to ask if they have any scars. The more open the pores of the skin are, the more vulnerable you are, a small intestine indicator. Acne indicates reabsorption of waste, long transit time, constipation, polycystic ovaries.

Note the location of any mole and the corresponding organ. Photograph the marking and watch for changes.

"The pathological face" as drawn by Matthew Wood and redrawn by Kay Parent.

138 AN INTRODUCTION TO *THE PRACTICING HERBALIST*

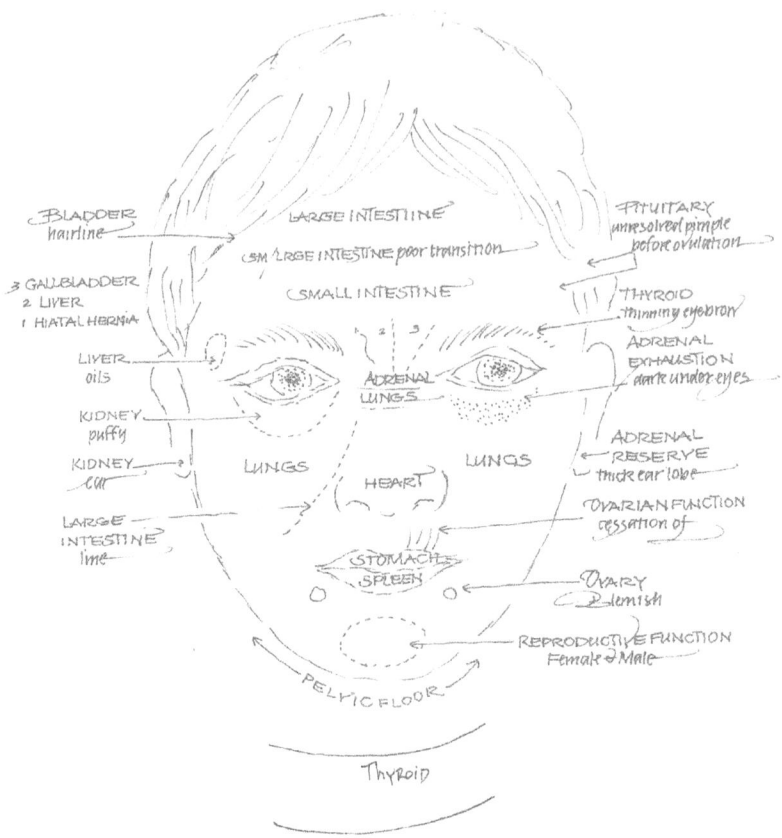

The following table summarizes conditions that can be observed through general facial analysis:

Facial indicator or area	Association
Hairline	Bladder/kidney
Face pale	Weakness, depletion, anemia. Blood not in stomach or spleen
Face puffy	Stagnation
FOREHEAD Upper	Large intestine
Lower	Small intestine

(Continued)

(Continued)

Facial indicator or area		Association
	Lines to one side	Problem is on that side. W.Le.
	Chopped up lines	Gut stress, colitis, irritable bowel
	Wiggly horizontal lines	Too much thinking, small intestine. "Dwelling on the past." Spleen, stomach
SIDE of HEAD	Edge of ear to eyebrow, the indent	Feel the area to feel the quality of the oil coming from the liver. Rough with pimples are gallstones. Spleen
	Left side, one inch inside hair line, bump that feels like a pimple with no head	Pituitary
CHEEKS		Lungs
	Diagonal line from large intestine line toward center of eye	Gravity line. The day, at a certain age, when tissues relax and reach for the Earth
EYES	Under eyes, puffy	Kidneys
	Under eyes, puffy outer crest of socket	Food allergies
	Under eyes, brown coloration	Liver
	Under eyes, blue–black coloration	Liver, adrenal, allergy
	Under eyes, blue puffy rectangle, outer eye socket orbit	Acute pain
	Wiggly vertical line between eyes	Hiatal hernia, tension in solar plexus, tightness across chest
	Horizontal line, midline between eyes	Adrenals. Coffee drinkers
	Vertical lines, to edges of eyes	Gallbladder

(Continued)

(Continued)

Facial indicator or area		Association
	Wiggly vertical lines outside eyes, running down outer cheek	Spleen, stomach weakness
	Horizontal lines between eyes	Asthma, holding breath
	Outside, pale blue, puffy rectangle	Intense pain
NOSE	Central	Stomach/lungs
	Tip	Heart
EARS	Red	High blood pressure
	Diagonal crease in lobe	Collapsed capillary bed, heart problem, most often associated with dehydration in uterus, liver (all are endocrine-functioning organs)
DEEP FURROW	From inner eye, curving along cheekbone	Large intestine. Habitual laxative use (coffee). Firm hard line, puffy, that may fork at end, may be toxic pathology if line rejoins (an island in the colon)
	Forked line, deeper at V	Has had surgery
	Drooping line along cheekbone	Sagging large intestine
	Feathered line along cheekbone	Atonic, weak
	Blackheads, with purple coloration of furrow	Stagnation
Pencil lips		Contraction
Lower lip		Intestines. Central red crack = ulcer. Blue–red is deep fever. M.W.

(Continued)

EXAMINING THE FACE 141

(Continued)

Facial indicator or area	Association
Jaw line	The pelvic floor. Look to the area of an eruption in relation to the area of the pelvis. Look to dental abscess/infection as the cause of systemic or specific pelvic infection
Temporal mandibular joint clenched, unmoving	Look to hips. Calcium deficiency
Neck Double rings, one above thyroid, one below	Early warning of longstanding thyroid imbalance
Large bulge over thyroid, sometimes to side	Goiter (thyroid)
Hard pea to larger lump on esophagus near thyroid	Nodule on thyroid
Other body associations	
Longer toe beside big toe	Lack of intrinsic factor
Hiatal hernia	Ileocecal valve
Dry skin, bumps on backs of arms	Omega 3 oil and calcium-deficient
Sheets of red bumps front of arms	Cold trapped under the skin

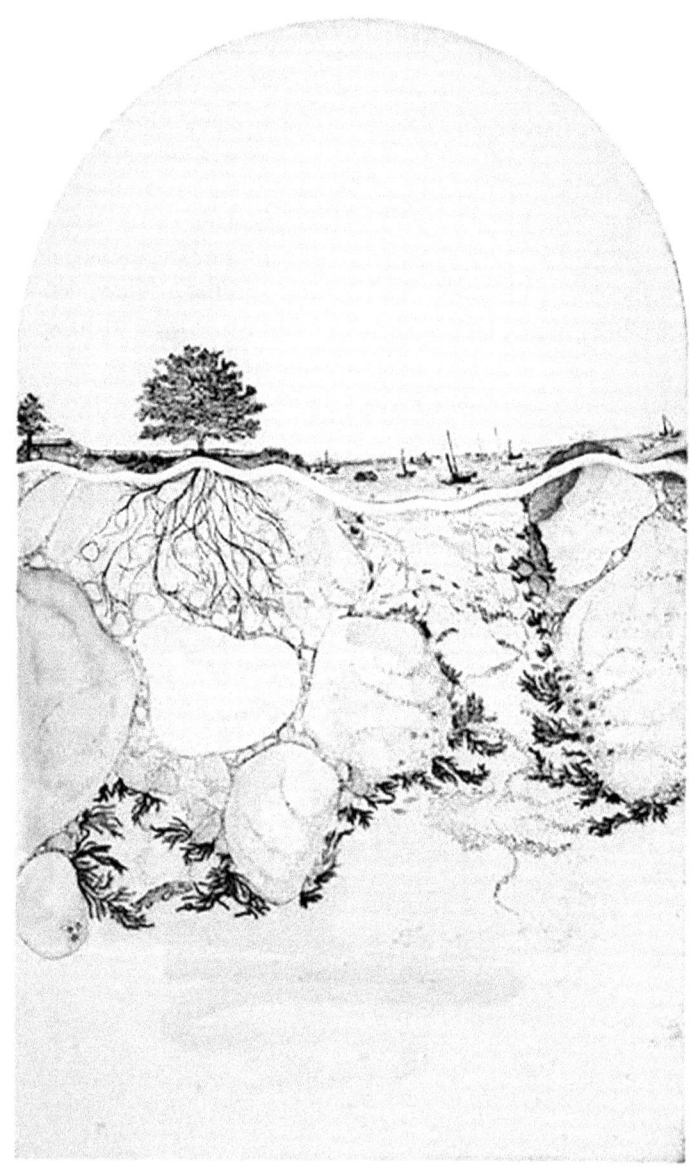

Late august

CHAPTER 10

Examining the eyebrows

Ask "Do you/did you pluck your eyebrows?" They often do not grow back.

The following table summarizes associations with eyebrows:

Eyebrow description	Association
Full and bushy right across	Good recuperative powers, strong ancestry. High androgen. P.D.L. Best constitution
Thin and delicate	Weaker constitution

(Continued)

(Continued)

Eyebrow description	Association
Choppy	Constitutional diseases. Hypothyroid
Dandruff	Allergies at the adrenal level
Outer eyebrow thinning	Hypothyroid imbalance

Compliment your client who has thick, bushy eyebrows. "You have a strong constitution!"

CHAPTER 11

Examining the eyes

Before evaluating ask: "Have you been in swimming pools, do you wear contacts, take medications, smoke, have allergies?"

General eye condition

The following table summarizes conditions that can be indicated by general eye conditions:

Eye description	Association
Floaters in eyes. These are floaters that the person sees in their vision	Liver, gallbladder, general eye problems, poor metabolism of fats
Bulging eyes	Look to hyperthyroid. "Looks like a hunted animal" Lycopus. M.W.
Mucus in eyes	Bacterial build-up. Rosemary eyewash (Graf). Goldenseal, Eyebright. M.W.

(Continued)

(Continued)

Eye description	Association
Weeping or running eyes	Weak kidneys. Sumac or other astringent. M.W. Allergies
Conjunctivitis. Big red splotches	Generalized redness with allergies (Goldenrod). Bloodshot (Ambrosia Ragweed). Nicole Telkes
Eye sand	Pineal gland
Crust where lashes meet lid	Lyme disease
Eyelashes crossing	Parasites. Lyme disease
Eyes water	Lack of oils or waters
Eyes can't focus	Growth of fibrin, hardening of eyeball. Liver, Lyme

Eye sockets

The area under the eyes (eyes socket) is the only part of the skin that does not sweat. Therefore, it shows the condition of the kidneys.

A half circle under the eye, only partway, is less serious. If a condition extends past the mid-point, the dividing line, it is a more serious liver issue. If it's halfway you have very good chances of having pretty quick results. "If the line goes further across, you're just going to have to work longer with them." Kay Parent. When people ask: "How long will I have to consume my formula?" Nose to one quarter under = 3 months, to mid-way = 6 months, three quarters = 9 months, and all the way to the far side of the eye = a year or longer.

The following table summarizes associations with conditions under the eyes:

Color/condition	Association
Distance of indication	Indication traveling past the center line is more serious. Longer recuperation
Puffy bags under eyes	Kidney/bladder weakness, edema (Nettles, Parsley)
Black	Adrenal exhaustion (Ginseng, Licorice, Siberian Eleuthero, Spikenard, Aralia racemosa). W.Le. Spikenard for "The journey too long." M.W.
Black line following socket	Specific food allergy. D.W.
Crosshatching	Diverticulitis
Dark, cross-hatched wrinkles; look to butt pimples, foot odor, toenail fungus	Toxic lymph fluids, stagnation in kidney, toxic colon
Puffy with brown coloration	Toxic lymph fluids, skin tags over lymphatic areas, stagnation in kidney, toxic colon

(*Continued*)

(Continued)

Color/condition	Association
Drooping bag beneath	Turbidity and edema in extremities. M.W.
Brown	Adrenal or kidney weakness (Teasel, Sarsaparilla)
Puffy, brown-washed, darkness under the eyes	Sinus infection or bronchitis
Brown wash, sepia	Stagnation of liver (Dandelion)
Orange, raised patches	Not assimilating Vitamin A, carotenoids
Red swelling beneath eye, above orbit	Allergies. With ADHD use Hawthorn. Look to lack of intrinsic factor
Red/pink -histamine/ autoimmune excess	Dark red—Dandelion. Infection to the bone
Gray–black or bluish	Prone to low BP, stagnation, water retention, coldness

(Continued)

(Continued)

Color/condition	Association
Yellow	Liver, gallbladder (Oregon Grape root, Balmony, Fringe Tree bark)
Yellow around eyes, red cheeks	Yellow dock. M.W.
Emaciating around the eyes, eyes becoming nervous and alert	"Drain on system" from chronic disease, indicating silica-containing remedies. (Avena, Equisetum, Couchgrass). M.W. From Eli Jones.
Dry beneath eye	Fluids depleted. Fluids depleted in lungs, use American Ginseng. M.W. Dry beneath with insecurity, use American Spikenard *Aralia*. M.W.
Sharp dark blackish-bluish color	Low in iron, usually pale face. Pain and cramps
Rut-like, sunken	Long-standing exhaustion
Blue with slight black. Caved in, sunken, translucent	Mild adrenal exhaustion. Up too late, studying too hard, kids in boarding school or college, lack of sleep, worrying while sleeping. Sleep is the main remedy
Blue, puffy "moonstone" rectangle at outer eye orbit 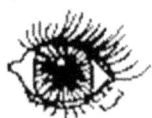	Acute pain

(*Continued*)

(Continued)

Color/condition	Association
White of eyeball showing beneath iris 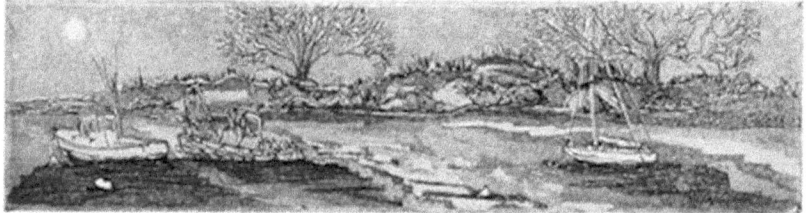	Deficient, may consume too much sugar or junk food

November nights

CHAPTER 12

Examining the sclera

Color of sclera

The study of sclerology, the study of the red lines in the sclera, was taught by Dr. Sundance, a Native American medicine man in Idaho, to Dori Denton ND and later used by William LeSassier.

"Below the sclera, broken blood vessels equal the digestive triangle." W.Le.

The following table summarizes conditions that can be indicated by the color of the sclera:

Color	Association
Pale blue	Anemia, poor circulation, nutrient and oxygen depletion
Blue in whites of eyes	Lack of oxygen
Yellow	Kidney/bladder weakness, edema (Nettles, Parsley)
Yellow–brown	Liver
Greenish	Gallbladder, poor bile formation

(Continued)

(Continued)

Color	Association
Red	Excessive heat, "reckless blood"; inflammation of liver, stomach, colon. The inner sclera especially indicate colon congestion
Red at edges	Some blood in some organs
Purplish tint	Mononucleosis
Pasty, off-white	Excess mucus, lymphatic congestion
White spaces, red veins	Carbon monoxide poisoning
Gray	Poor elimination, constipation, sluggish bowel

Pupils

Pupils should dilate under light and respond evenly. William said: "The iris is the primary way of substantiating issues." He turned to the iris when he couldn't find the issue elsewhere.

The following table summarizes associations with pupil conditions:

Pupil condition	Association
Contracting/dilating	Weak adrenals, hypothalamus. Vata. (Ginseng, Licorice)
Extreme contraction (miosis)	Disease of spinal cord or nervous system disorders. Heat, contraction. Pitta
Extreme dilation (mydriasis)	Epilepsy, severe anemia, TB, LSD use, irritation of nervous system. Kapha. Lack of enervation from low blood sugar
Uneven right to left pupil	Head injury, MS, sarcoidosis

"When you give the right remedy, very often the eyes shine. Watch for it." M.W.

Client's view

Gray amorphic floaters, the bacterial life of the eyeball

Light spots	Anemia
Reduction in clarity	Fibrous tissue growth, cataracts, glaucoma, diabetes, a night of drinking

Below eyelid

This is an old medical technique refined by William LeSassier. Have the client pull the lower eyelid down and look up; a small half-moon is exposed inside the eyelid, the palpebral conjunctiva.

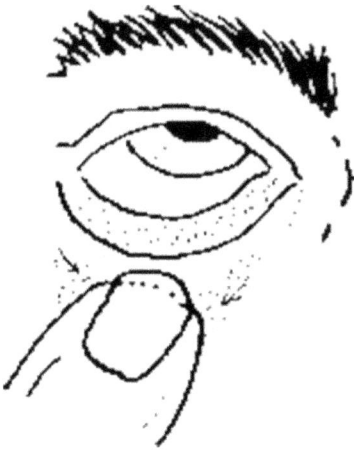

The following table summarizes indications associated with conditions below the eyelid:

Condition below eyelid	Indication
All evenly pink	Healthy
Areas of white	Anemia. Lack of circulation. Look to paleness of face, lips, fingernail beds
Central white	Center of body, blood deficiency in uterus. Paler toward the center is a deep anemia. Paler toward the outside is a shallow anemia

(*Continued*)

(Continued)

Condition below eyelid	Indication
Areas of red	Heat
Conjunctivitis	Contagious eye infection. Eye wash with strained Goldenseal. Black tea bag poultices. Wash all doorknobs and pens, steering wheel with rubbing alcohol

Eyelid

Stye	Infected follicle, too much thinking. Spleen or pancreas
Upper eyelid droops, decreasing vision	Muscle atrophy, genetic? Hypothyroid? Lack of intrinsic factor?
Blepharitis	Blocked follicle, builtup sebum within eyelid

EXAMINING THE SCLERA 155

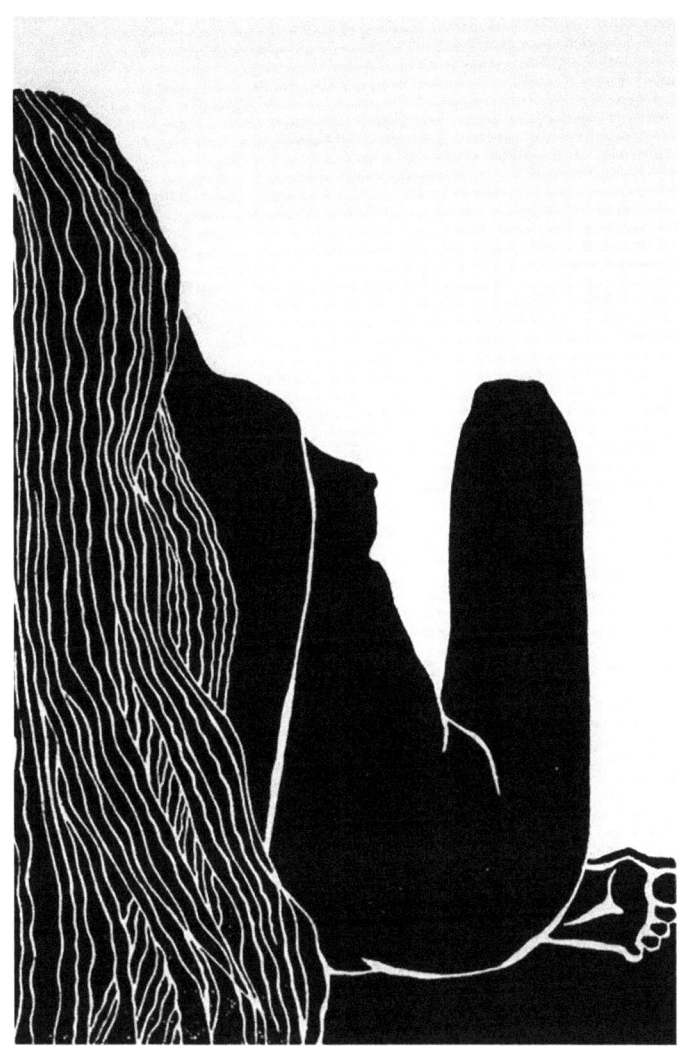

Dreamed self portrait

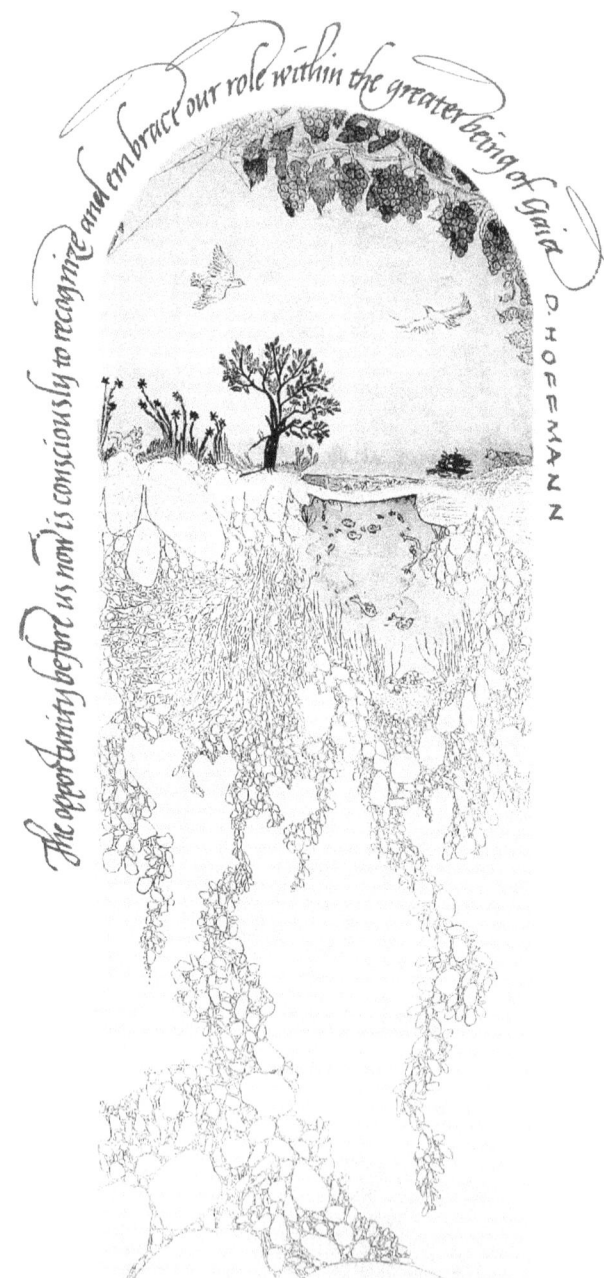

Sunset pond with calligraphy

CHAPTER 13

Examining the nose

The nose indicates heart, lungs, digestion, and the element of metal. Look to the shape of the nostrils and the development of the nose. All nostrils differ in size. Noses are air places. They're supposed to let air in and keep particulate matter out. Lots of hair in a nose—good job! Heart is a reflection of the lifestyle.

The following table summarizes nose characteristics and associations:

Nose description	Association
An uncomplicated nose The Porky Pig nose, two circles and a knob	Fewer problems
A long, thin, elaborate arabesque nose	More sensitive. Tends to have allergies, more food sensitivities. The thinner the nose, the greater the problems

(Continued)

(Continued)

Nose description	Association
Tip red, swollen, square, or white	Heart problems
Red, swollen, bulbous	Alcoholism, rosacea
Red, chapped nostrils at the interface of inside and outside the nose	Inflammation of stomach Food allergies Look to lack of intrinsic factor
Line across nose	Allergies. Large intestine
Corners of nose	Large intestine
Crevice at the side of nose with bluish veins	Pelvic floor, hemorrhoids
Crevice with blackheads	Large intestine reabsorbing toxins
Tip looks like it was cut off and put back on	Heart problems
Irregular, slightly misshapen in one quadrant "Always this way or a change?"	Valve problem, slightly enlarged heart Deviated septum of nose. P.D.L.
Polyps? Inflamed adenoids? Uvula malformation?	Strained breathing, breathing through mouth. Ask about Apnea	Try sea vegetables!

CHAPTER 14

Examining the teeth, mouth, and lips

Specific indications of the teeth and gums

The following table describes specific tooth indications:

"Chaotic teeth" W.Le.	Internal strife in early life. Lack of Vitamin A in the womb. P.D.L. Vata
Perfectly aligned teeth	Pitta
Cavities abundant	Lack of calcium. Use 1 teaspoon Horsetail *Equisetum hyemale* daily, powdered, take 6 days off and repeat. Doug Simons
Grinding teeth	Parasites, lack of calcium
Much tooth decay with a dry tongue	Lack of saliva to protect the teeth, yin deficiency. Christopher Hobbs. Use American Ginseng
Jaw pain, deep in the bone	Decalcification. Use 1 teaspoon Horsetail *Equisetum hyemale* daily, powdered, take 6 days off and repeat. Doug Simons. Medical testing if persists
Receding gums	Liver deficiency. D. Simons
Gum wounds	Agrimony aerial parts. Christopher Hedley
Toothache	Yarrow root. Christopher Hedley

Crooked teeth indicate "Poor digestive upbringing." William LeSassier.

> Doug Simons sat cross-legged under his wide straw hat, New Mexican sun and earth, our classroom, he shared many new thoughts. "Toothpaste is made with glycerin. Glycerin makes your teeth look shiny and feel smooth. Pretty. Glycerin stops the production of Amylase and impedes the production of saliva. Amylase and saliva are needed to avoid cavities and maintain healthy digestion!"

Teeth need opposing pressure. Try Black Willow twigs, snap them to create a chisel edge and firmly press against teeth, drawing the stick from gum to tip. "It takes about three strokes a tooth, which sounds like a lot of time, but actually takes the same amount of time as responsible tooth brushing. You simply press and drag, it feels great and gives you something constructive to do in the car. Then massage your gums down toward the tips of teeth and back into place." No more receding gums! Doug views receding gums as a liver deficiency and recommends bitters prior to meals—a few drops of tincture into water.

Doug uses Red Root and Chaparral tea to rinse the mouth with whenever there are painful teeth. "Eat Garlic and Greens."

Examining the mouth

A normal mouth will have a lip above that has a little definition. An equal size above and below is healthy, less troubled with digestive issues. It means you're not deficient in any particular area. W.Le.

Upper duodenum Pyloric valve left side Lower duodenum	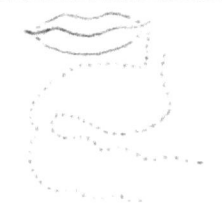
Cracks or ulcers at corners of mouth enzyme deficiency B vitamin deficiency Vitamin B-2 deficiency. Ulcerative colitis	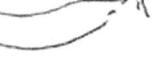

(Continued)

(Continued)

Lines from edges of mouth to chin On the person Right line is duodenum Left is pyloric and ileocecal valves	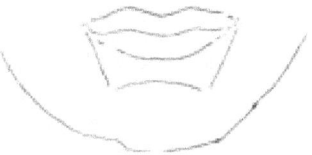

Lips

The following table summarizes mouth and lip characteristics and associations:

Mouth/lip description	Association
Simple lip, equal in proportion	Fewest of digestive problems. They tend to have really great constitutions and can eat anything
Fussy lip, Batman lips	More trouble digesting
Small upper lip	Carbohydrates okay. M.W.
Corners turn down	Makes digestion unhappy. Liver Chi stagnation. W.Le. Vata, stress. P.D.L.
Drooping	Lyme disease, palsy, forceps birth
Cracks and dryness	B-vitamin deficiency, fatty acid deficiency, yin deficiency, irritation, dryness. D.W.

(Continued)

(Continued)

Mouth/lip description	Association
Central crack down the center	Irritation from gastric juices. History of ulcer
Chapped lower lip	Lack of spleen and pancreas function. Dehydration
Mouth open all the time	Poor digestion, sinus blockage, swollen tissues. People who always have their mouth open usually have poor digestion from swallowing a lot of air with food and while talking
Dark outlining of the lips	Excess melanin production, hormonal imbalance. Look to the pineal gland
Dry cracked lips, coated tongue	Stagnant heat, fermenting
Inside lips blue Inside lips angry red	Lack of oxygen to center. High blood pressure, ulcer, cardiac issue, gastritis. W.Le.

CHAPTER 15

Examining the chin

"When examining the chin, move it around, and check for adhesions." TMJ down around the chin corresponds to the pelvic floor.

The following table summarizes chin characteristics and associations. All are from William unless otherwise noted.

Chin description		Association
Small chin in relation to the rest of the face		Low libido, weak water element
Large chin in relation to the rest of the face		Strong libido, strong constitution for digestion
Dimple		Not so strong libido and constitution. Possible heart murmur

(*Continued*)

(Continued)

Chin description	Association
Cleft	Driven by reproductive organs. Strong
Pimples over ovary points	Cyst, fibroid or tumor
Irregular lumpy tissue in the chin, palpate with fingers	Toxins and lumps in the pelvic region
Pimple on one side	Ovary on that side
Whole area breaks out	Lymph system in pelvic floor. Polycystic ovary syndrome, multiple follicular cysts
Lines, broken or wiggly, from lip corners to chin	Small intestine spasticity
Changes in texture, color, or lines, outbreaks of any kind. Constant touching	Prostate, testes issues
With red rashes	Indicates heat, inflammation

Examining beneath the chin

Brown pigment, skin tags	Toxicity of the lymphatics beneath

CHAPTER 16

Examining the tongue

A healthy tongue is pink and evenly coated, with a light-rooted coating. There could be a straight central line, the primary fold from birth, with no crevasses, indentations, or marks. The tongue sticks straight out easily so that you can see two-thirds of it and it does not shake. Big bumps on the back of the tongue are normal, fungiform papillae. Mushroom-like. Hold the tongue out for 15 seconds and rest.

William LeSassier intoned: "The tongue should protrude easily, be moist, red and inviting."

Tongue scraping is great; it rids the body of bacteria and toxins. A tongue scraper is a stainless-steel U-shaped device. You place it at the back of the tongue and scrape forward. All of the toxins from your night of cleansing during sleep are pulled forward and dumped into the sink. Easy. You can boil it occasionally or throw it into the dishwasher. Don't ever brush your tongue with the toothbrush. All the bacteria are lodged into the filaments, and they grow and multiply to join you the next time you brush. Disgusting. Recent medical tests indicate that daily tongue scraping reduces bacterial throat infections up to 60 percent. Scraping cleanses the bloodstream and increases Chi. Nice.

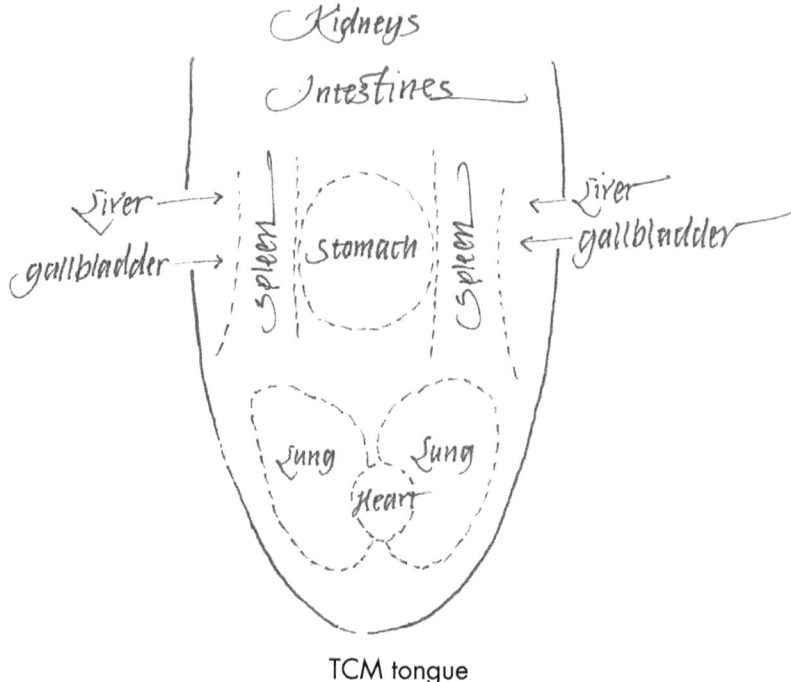

TCM tongue

LeSassier tongue diagram

The following table describes areas of the tongue and their relationship to areas of the body:

Area of the tongue	Area of the body
Whole tongue	Heart
Back—swollen red fungiform papillae	Old infections in bloodstream
Back left	Kidney
Back central	Large intestine
Central line wiggle	Scoliosis/vertebrae out
Central line	Spine/digestive tube endocrine system
Central line, cross-hatched	Cross-hatching may indicate pathology
Center line, curve toward side	Hiatal hernia
Back right	Uterus

(Continued)

EXAMINING THE TONGUE

(Continued)

Area of the tongue	Area of the body
Central left	Liver
Central rear	Small intestine
Central right	Gallbladder
Center	Stomach/spleen
Central front	Lung
Edges	Blood stream, lymphatics, overall stress level
Angry-colored fissure	Possible pathology
Edges, lines	Breast changes
Tip	Throat, sinuses, mind

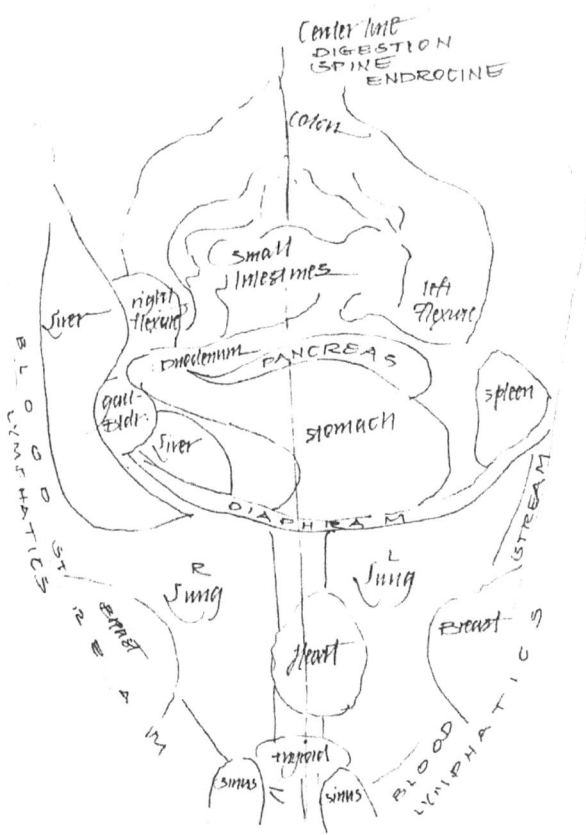

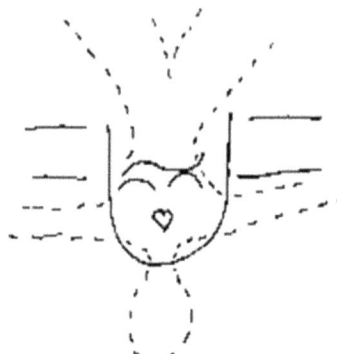

Tongue body, literally

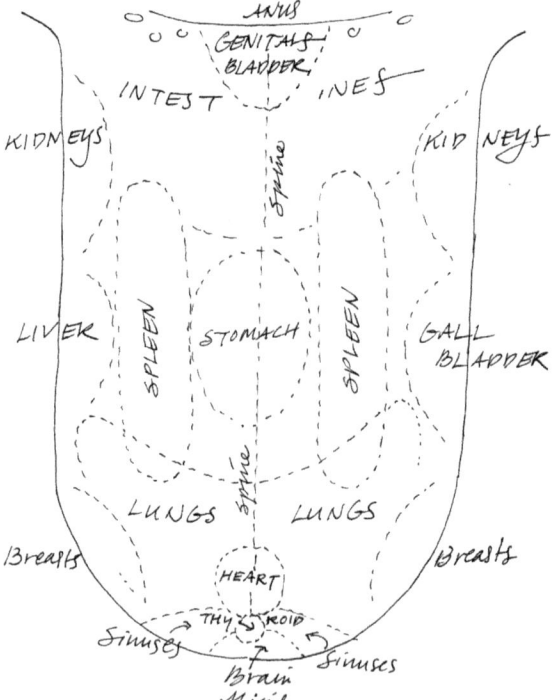

The Heart organ is indicated. The Heart more broadly includes the thyroid and mind. The spine line is sometimes congenital and sometimes indicates gastrointestinal.

Matthew Wood tongue

The spirit of the tongue

Vata	Pitta	Kapha
"Medium long, thin and dry"	"Flame-like, reddish, elongated"	Round, full, damp, pale, short
Elongated or thin and like a taut muscle. Withered	Matthew Wood after Christopher Hobbs	

The following table summarizes the conditions that can be indicated through general tongue analysis:

Overall tongue condition	Association
Easily comes out, even light red color, even rooted coating, stationary, strong, moist. M.W.	Healthy
Branched line	Two or more organs affected by a common cause. W.Le.
Prolapsed dome	Atonic or prolapsed condition. W.Le.
Domed, swollen, or wet area	Stagnation, weak, atonic tissue. W.Le.
Chained lines	Chronic weakness, longstanding infections. W.Le.

(Continued)

170   AN INTRODUCTION TO *THE PRACTICING HERBALIST*

(Continued)

Overall tongue condition	*Association*
Island	Area that has been scarred or healed broken bone. W.Le.
Jagged lines	Sudden or acute infection having damaged that organ. W.Le.

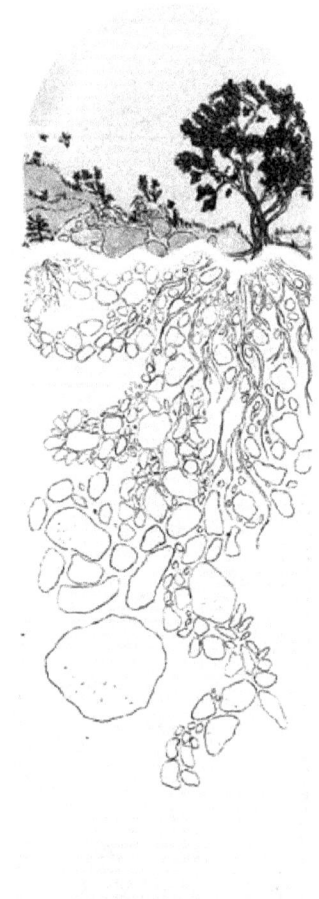

Pathway

Specific tongue indications

When using tongue analysis to assess issues, look to the nails and forehead for confirmation. "Clean the lungs in the fall, the liver in the spring." W.Le. "Tongue is the outer expression of stomach Chi." W.M. The following table describes specific tongue indications:

Overall tongue condition	Association
Pale	Cold, blood and Chi deficient, menses
Flaccid	Atonic, weak
Swollen tongue, domed	Tissue swelling in that organ Edema, spleen If red, excess heart fire; if pale, excess cold or damp
Trembles, shakes	Adrenal exhaustion, low blood sugar or lethargic, weak. Liver wind-spasticity. D.W. Look to pupils for contracting and dilating, trembling hands. Hyperadrenalism
Central red	Heat in the stomach, intestines, spleen The more red toward the tip indicates severe upper burner heat
Geographic or mapped tongue	Phlegm fire, heat baking down fluids, thickened fluids blocking heat. "Dark, red tongue tissue covered by thick white or sometimes yellow coating, ripped off in patches. Always Dandelion!" M.W. "Poor digestive upbringing. Parasites."

(Continued)

(Continued)

Overall tongue condition	Association
Frothy streamers down sides	Look to lungs. Shallow breathing. Dampness in spleen issuing out through intestines or lungs
Coating over tip	Mental confusion

Characteristic	Association
Ruts in front	Past or present lung weakness, asthma, pneumonia. Ask if they bit their tongue, a scar
Curved lines at edge	Spleen deficiency, tons of gas. Dry digestion. Vata. Enzyme issues. W.M.
Pointy red tongue tip	Excess HCl or heat in the digestive tract. Pitta. Heart heat
Scalloped edges	B vitamin deficiency, weak "spleen," small intestine. (Gentian, Ginseng.) Look to nails, forehead. "Too much worry." Ulcers in the scallops? Goldenseal. M.W.

(Continued)

(Continued)

Characteristic	Association
Glossy, mirror-like	Hot flashes, night sweats. W.M. Not holding onto nutrients.
Central line	Spinal column, digestive system, endocrine system
Hollow rut, sides curl up	Deficient
Wiggle of central line at tip	Neck
Central line, chained, phlegm in stomach area	B-12 deficiency. Historical amount of worry and aggravation Yarrow
Curved line at first third	Diaphragm significance. M.W.
Central line across middle	Diaphragm tension

(Continued)

(Continued)

Characteristic	Association
Diaphragm area has a wiggle like an S	Hiatal hernia
Central line angry red, raw, deep with yellowish mucus	Ulcer, pre-ulcer. Heat in digestive tract Stress Yarrow. M.W.
Cracks down the center, wiggly lines to the side	Lack of assimilation. Look to nails, forehead More crossing, redness and depth, the more pathology and heat (Catnip, Yarrow)
Small, angular, criss-crossing on back third	Bowel pockets Irritation of bowel, diverticulitis Slippery Elm, Yarrow
Criss-crossing (as above) with red in the cracks	Heat in the digestive tract. Diverticulitis (Slippery Elm, Marshmallow) Look to nails, forehead (Yarrow)
Big, white, and pasty	Hypothyroid
Puffy and pale	Atonic organs, weak heart, edema Kidney weakness

(Continued)

(Continued)

Characteristic	Association
Froth on edges, bubbles Frothy streamers	Look to lungs, shallow breathing Dampness in spleen. Issuing out through intestines or lungs
Flat, wide tongue	Organs have grown larger—high altitudes
Twisted tongue	Scoliosis, MS, polio. Dyslexia Front is upper spine, mid is mid-spine, back is lower spine
Crooked tongue	Liver wind, stroke, cranial nerve XII damage Perhaps from forceps used at birth
Canker sores on tongue	Ulcers in digestive tract (Melissa, Horsetail, Sage, Agrimony, Raspberry) Systemic over-acidity, herpes or syphilis, heat in upper burner (Melissa, Horsetail, Goldthread, St. John's Wort)

Deep furrows
  tip = lungs
  middle = stomach
  sides = liver (serious)
  back sides = kidneys "really" M.W.
	Dehydration, poor electrolyte balance
	Ask if they have water filtration, which removes all minerals. Eat seaweed

(Continued)

(Continued)

Characteristic	Association
Chopped hamburger meat	Cancer. As the cancer progresses it looks as though a cleaver cut the meat many times. Eli Jones. Ground Ivy
Tooth marks on one or both sides	Bronchial issue in past; pneumonia, bronchitis as a child
Slit at tip, double tooth marks	Tonsils out
Sides cracked Angry red or white patches that do not scrape	Breast changes, lymphatics May be pathology
Under tongue, stalagtite-like growths growing down from the bottom	Serious vitamin B deficiency. B-12 Inappropriate fat and cholesterol issues Definite lack of intrinsic factor! Needs only this indication to require methyl-cobalamin
Crack down the middle, opening up	Heat in digestive tract Yarrow likely. M.W.
Blue veins under upturned tongue (sublingual engorgement) Blue/purple/dry Varicose blue	Blood stagnation, varicose veins, pelvic floor stagnation Internal heat or external cold. W.M. Exuberant heat/depletion of fluids Cyanotic

(Continued)

EXAMINING THE TONGUE

(Continued)

Characteristic	Association
Crack down the middle, opening up to reveal crossed cracks	Yarrow
Red edges	Heat in liver or gallbladder rising to head with wind creating anger, liver fire. Liver time. M.W. If only red at tip is heart fire or sinuses
Contracted tongue, barely reaches beyond the teeth	Wasting disease, heart, blood deficiency. Many years on earth
"Withered"	Nutritional deficiency
Withdrawn, cannot get it out	Severely deficient, possible nerve damage. Elder years
With green coloration and moist	Cold, stiffening of muscles, vessels, tendons. Dehydrated and cold—stiff muscles and tendons
Withered and swollen	Mucous and dampness have accumulated inside the organ
Plus pink and dry	Impairment of body fluids by heat
Stiff, hard	Heat contraction, pain
Withered, purple	Heart deficiency, nutritional deficiency

Coating on the tongue

Tongue coatings give clues to the overall state of the person. An even, light, rooted coating of mucus on the tongue is healthy. A rooted coating is one that doesn't scrape off.

The following table describes indications associated with tongue coating:

Coating description	Association
Thick coating	Candida, phlegm, Kapha, mucus
Greasy	Phlegm, dampness, stagnation; gas, indigestion. Gallbladder Use alteratives
Yellow coating	Heat. Liver or gallbladder, look to location. Large intestine: do they have constipation, dry hard stools? Inflammation of stomach area (with red irritated surface, ulcer). (Licorice, Slippery Elm, Comfrey) Alteratives likely
Light yellow/greasy and slippery, like an oil slick in streaks	Gallbladder. Too many fats in the diet, deficient liver/gallbladder function (Celandine)
Yellow–brown	Heat in the interior, constipation, liver/spleen, pancreas (Bupleurum, Oregon Grape root, Gentian, Dandelion). Putrid, septic
Orange	Spleen/pancreas (Turmeric, Gentian, Dandelion)
Orange dot on right frontal section	Gallbladder. Without lifting head, first thing in the morning, hold a mirror up and you can see the dot
Gray coating on back third of the tongue	Sluggish bowel, constipation, smoking, and excess heat. (Stop smoking, drink fluids, eat soluble fiber, exercise). Use fresh ground Flax seeds, Slippery Elm, fresh fruits
Black (hairy with elongation of papillae)	Radiation treatment, fungal infection
Black coating on back third	Toxicity, possible degenerative condition, fungal infection, or bacterial infection, heat causing tissue death. (Echinacea, Baptisia). Can be normal in extreme age

(Continued)

(Continued)

Coating description	Association
Moist mucus	Excess bile, indigestion, poor organ activity, dampness (Wild Yam, mild Ginger tea)
Dry tongue, furred (like a damp cat with peaks of hair standing up)	They have secretions but they dry out. Excess heat, irritation, fever (Slippery Elm, nervines). Check area of tongue. Check skin—is it dry? If so, the whole system is dry. Increase fluids
Frothy mucus on edges	Look to lungs. Phlegm in lungs. Shallow breathing
"Strawberry tongue"	Classic indication for homeopathic Belladonna, especially in children's fevers
Smooth, like glass	No assimilation. Exhausted stomach, malnutrition. (Lemon juice in water, Sweetleaf *Monarda fistulosa*)
Raised red papillae on tongue	Systemic infection. (Echinacea, Calendula)
Purple–red	Engorged or stagnant heart. Look for puffiness of tongue, scalloped edges. (Hawthorn, Rosehips)
White	Cold fluid stagnation or excess secretion. Wild Geranium
Central forward area red, raw, coated	Ulcer

Specific papillae indications

I see all the filiform papillae from teeny red dots to large pale pink spots as representing an immune or lymph imbalance. Dots indicate heat coming from a deeper level up through the superficial tissues. The redder the dots are, the more active the inflammatory response. The more inactive pale, pink spots represent lymphatic stagnation.

The following table describes indications associated with tongue coating:

Papillae description	Indications	Papillae description	Indications
Small dots, tend to be toward tip. Allergies. M.W.	Allergic response: Look to red cheeks, red puffiness beneath eyes, inflammation. Hawthorn. M.F.	Raised red papillae on back third/center	Heat in intestines and urinary tract. Hemorrhoids, cystitis, urethritis Heat in spleen, stomach, intestines. W.Le.
Larger dots, tend toward mid and lower. M.W.	Swollen lymphatics Larger the dot the bigger the heat Mid to lower region = lymph	Raised red papillae all over	Systemic infection, septicemia, infection, heat in the blood (Echinacea, Baptisia)
Tiny dots on tongue body	Swollen glands, systemic infection. Immune challenge	Small red dots toward the tip	Allergies or irritability of the mucosa Heat in the heart
Red or pink papillae with dry tongue. M.W.	Peach leaf.	Dots toward the back of the tongue	Heat in the intestines
Pink spots up and down the sides of the tongue. M.W.	Old unresolved infections in the lymphatics. Calendula. M.W.	Dots at sides	Heat in liver and/or gallbladder

Thyroid tongue indications

Remember to look for two other indications, eyebrows thinning, neck rings, dull brittle nails and hair, dull thinking, weight changes, eyes bulging or droopy eyelids, calcium assimilation, blood sugar and digestive issues, plus broken blood vessels on the face.

Tongue appearance	Meaning
Divit toward tip, may be hollow or puffed	Hypothyroid
Redness near tip	Thyroid imbalance
Two lines near tip, sometimes an indentation or a raised area	Thyroid imbalance
Raised ball toward tip	Nodules on thyroid. Gently palpate thyroid—you may feel it
Divit at end of tongue, butt-like often red	Hyperthyroid

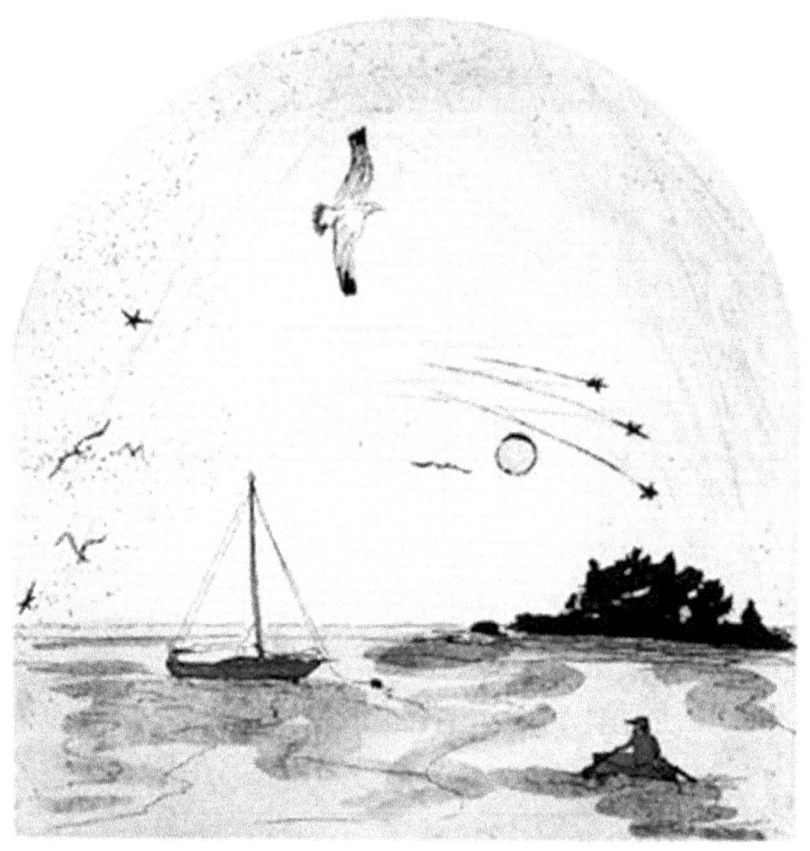
Shooting stars

CHAPTER 17

Examining the fingernails

The nail should fit nicely on the finger. The hand needs to be relaxed and below the level of the heart when you examine fingernails. Does client use polish (acetone poisoning) or buff the tops of the nails?

The more lunula—the white moons—the better a person's health is. Good circulation with many moons. It is said that moons from thumb to pinky indicate enough protein. Just to round things out, in Chinese medicine too many lunula indicates too yin.

The following table summarizes conditions that can be indicated by the condition or color of the fingernails:

Condition/color	Association
Ridges	Lack of assimilation. Chronic nervous system involvement. Hypothyroidism. Rheumatoid arthritis
Little skin flaps on sides of nails	Silica or Vitamin B deficiency

(Continued)

(Continued)

Condition/color	Association
Pale nail beds	Anemia. No blood to the surface "Have your period?" will be pale
Pale centers	Blood stagnating in center, uterus
Blue at base of nail by cuticle	Poor circulation and blood stagnation
Soft nails	Mineral deficient. Vitamin B deficiency. P.D.L.
Spongy, barely attached	TB, bronchitis, cancer, starts on index finger. Emphysema, look for blue color. Cystic fibrosis
Dipped-in nail	Longstanding deficiency. Not enough spirit time, relaxation. Meditate
Nail turns up	Asthma, misuse of adrenal sprays. Starts on index finger
Brittle	Thyroid condition, kidney, circulation iron deficiency. Vata
Black bits under the nail	Infectious endocarditis, serious heart infection, bleeding disorder (mitral valve prolapse, having teeth cleaned) Fungus

(Continued)

(Continued)

Condition/color	Association
Spoon-shaped or dark nails	Vitamin B-12 deficiency, cleaning with bleach reaction, anemia. Heart enlargement, look to other heart issues. Lead poisoning. D.W.
Flat nails	Deficiency. Raynaud's disease. Look to liver
Pitted red–brown spots, frayed and split ends	Psoriasis. Need Vitamin C, folic acid, and protein
Nail fungus	Overall alkalinity of sweat and body tissues
Long thick white mark, furrow across nail	Serious surgery
Red line at edge of nail, and cuticle	Blood caught in the extremities. Systemic connective tissue disorder, Lupus, nail biting
Reddish brown line	Kidneys. P.D.L.
Red/brown lines on cuticles	Heat or old infection. Misuse of antibiotics
White	Anemia, cold hands and feet. Raynaud's. (Safflower). M.W. "No blood to the surface." W.Le.
Horizontal ridges	Interference with life force. Systemic depletion. Too much Chlorine in the water system. P.D.L.

(Continued)

(Continued)

Condition/color	Association
Very red	Heat in the system
Weak nails, bites nails, hangnails	Silica deficiency (Avena, Equisetum)
Yellow nails and elevation of nail tips	Internal disorders may show here first. Lymphatic, respiratory, diabetes, liver
Thick nails	Poor blood circulation. May be thyroid. Fungus
Spots on nails	Big cloud? Ask: "Did you hit that nail?" Calcium-deficient is a large dull cloud. (Ask about bone loss, cavities, grinding teeth). How long to grow out? Bright tight spot? Zinc: ask if they have a poor sense of smell or poor tissue healing
Lunula over 1/3 nail	Weak constitution

(Continued)

(Continued)

Condition/color	Association
Curls downward	Blood deficiency, lung deficiency, chronic cough
Ridges, rounding and horizontal	Malnutrition. V. Lad
Transverse groove	Chronic fever, longstanding illness. V. Lad
White line, horizontal	Arsenic poisoning. D.W.
Half pink, half white	Kidney infection
Clubbing	Lung and liver. Heart, cyanotic heart disease, chronic pulmonary disease, cirrhosis, colitis

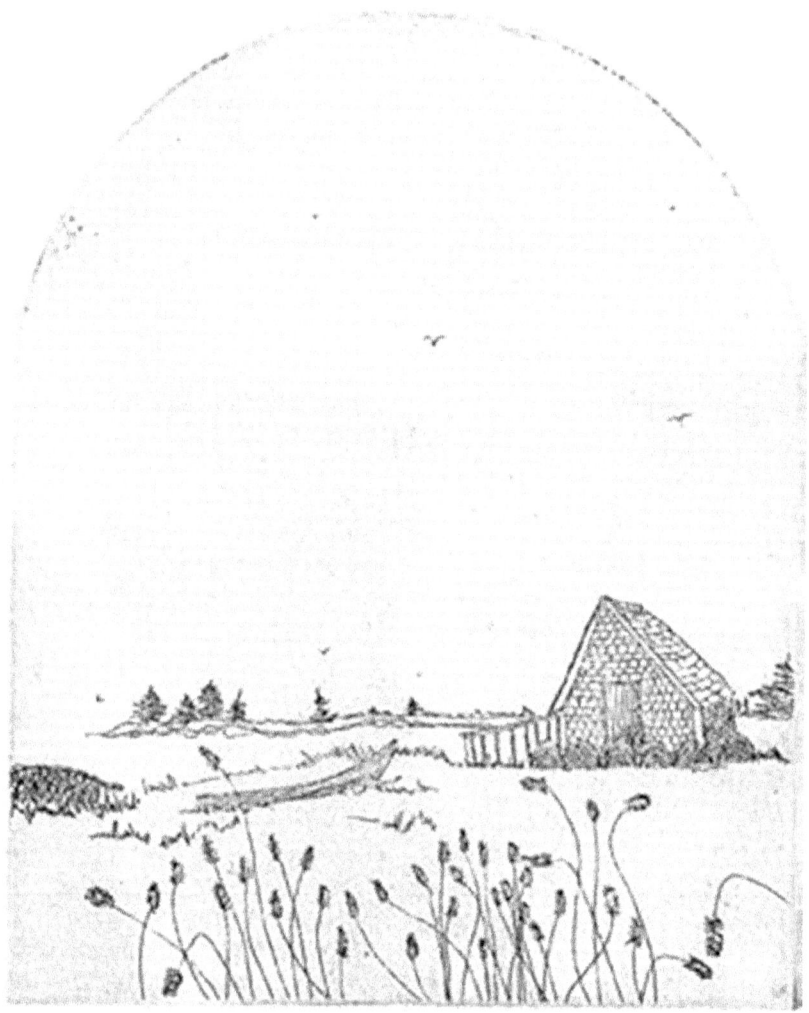

Fishing shed

CHAPTER 18

Examining the large intestine lines

The large intestine line follows the cheekbone, curving from near the inner eye socket to near the outer lip along the nose. The depth, pouching, forking, and shapes running along this line are all indicators of the tone, transit time, and vitality of the organ. The more droop along the cheek/nose line that forms a pouch, as though the tissue is a little bit plump and then it's hanging over, the more serious the issue.

The following table summarizes conditions indicated by examining large intestine lines:

Facial line	Diagram	Indication
Large intestine line		Early indication of sluggish elimination

(Continued)

(Continued)

Facial line	Indication
Blue coloration in line—pull cheek away from nose to note coloration	Lack of oxygenation, lack of blood circulation
Pimples in line	Toxicity, reabsorption of fecal matter
A feathered line	Delicate constitution, sensitive to foods and environment
A pouched line, plump, which droops over	Stagnation, diet low in fiber and/or rich in carbohydrates
A forked line	Scar from a polyp removed; it is as though it has created a pinch in the system. Scar from lesion, hemorrhoid, fissure
Forked line with opposite line or lines beginning to create a diamond shape	Stagnation in the large intestine caused by a blockage, tumor, prolapse. W.Le.
A diamond shape, and within the diamond is a puffy pouch. This is much more dramatic than a "plain" pouch.	"Pathology island" Schedule colonoscopy

Look to the upper forehead, base of skull headache, fingernails with ridges, skin outbreaks, candida, and tension in muscles.

Grab your Heart

— Rosemary

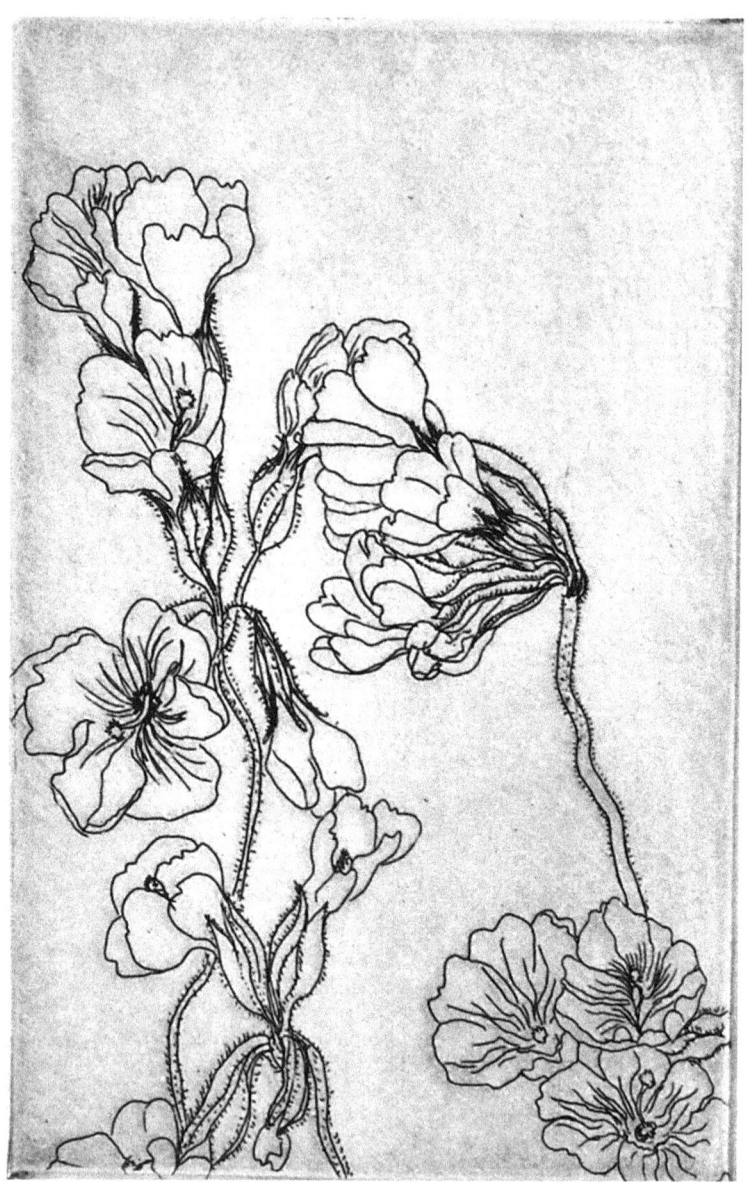

Swiss flowers

CHAPTER 19

Examining elimination

Stool analysis

Matt Wood and I had a discussion on this subject, at which time he took notes—and here they are:

> One herbalist who is not embarrassed to ask people about their intimate bodily functions is Margi Flint. Thus, she is an expert in diagnosis from the stool, as I found out while interviewing her at her busy office in Marble-head, MA. The "perfect bowel movement," says Margi, "is brown, about an inch or slightly more in diameter, a good seven inches to ten inches long, comes out perfectly when one is prompted to relieve oneself, moves easily and evenly when one sits down, forms a round curly-cue—like soft serve ice cream—slowly sinks to the bottom of the toilet gracefully and leaves one in a good mood." Deviations from this are evidence of disharmony manifesting in the digestive tract.

We look to seven factors in analyzing the stool: (1) transit time, (2) consistency, (3) color, (4) shape, (5) odor, (6) substances and worms, and (7) ease of passage.

Transit time

Healthy transit time is about six to twelve hours from the time of eating, depending on the food eaten. Fruit tends to shorten transit time, while meat, bread, and foods slow to digest lengthen transit time.

Eating cooked corn and waiting for it to pass can measure transit time. Look for the yellow kernel in the stool. "I got that one from Tieraona Low Dog," says Margi.

Slow transit time indicates difficulty in digesting meals, poor digestive secretion, poor tone of intestinal walls, and weak peristalsis. The stool tends to become hard and difficult to move.

Rapid transit time is indicated by undigested food in the stool, and non-absorption of water from the stool as it passes rapidly through the large intestine. The pores of the intestine are closed, resulting in incomplete uptake of water from the digestate. Symptoms are gurgling, excess gas, dampness in the stool, putrefaction, fermentation, infection, bloating, candida, and diarrhea. Stool is loose, unformed, and difficult to hold back. These conditions often call for Yellow Dock root *Rumex crispus*, Rhubarb *Rheum palmatum* or some member of the Polygonaceae family. M.W.

A stool that starts out hard and ends up loose indicates an untoned, unexercised colon, and a need for fiber.

Normal, healthy bowel movements usually occur shortly after rising from bed. Diarrhea sometimes drives people from bed in the morning. This is an indication for *Rumex crispus*. Delay of stool after rising indicates that transit time is slow. If coffee needs to be consumed before the passage, this is lack of tone. If a cigarette is necessary, this indicates self-medication for intestinal spasm—here consider Lobelia.

Basically, you put food in and it triggers a response to let the previously processed meal out. To poop three times a day is achieving "Colon-vana," says Matt Wood, smiling eyes fluttering.

Consistency

Hard stools indicate slow transit time, soft stools, fast transit time. Alternating hard and soft, constipation and diarrhea, indicates intestinal spasm and quirky peristalsis.

Stools that float contain air, mucus, fiber, or fat. A stool that floats and is well-shaped, textured and chocolate brown has enough fiber and is perfect.

    Stools that float, shred, and fall apart easily are full of air. Generally, these people swallow air while eating. If this is pointed out to them, they can correct their habit. Air can also indicate fermentation. A stool coated with mucus floats and is loose (three times a day or more often), indicating colitis.

    If there are food parts evident in the stool, then the digestive tract is not breaking down food. Such people need to chew more fully and perhaps take enzymes. In the case of diarrhea, the tract does not have enough time to break down the stool, hence it is moist and sometimes contains food.

Color

Iron supplements cause the stool to become artificially dark. Dark black stool indicates typhoid. Moderately dark color means not enough water and fiber and too much heavy food that is hard to digest. The stool is concentrated and tends to dry out into round, hard fecal balls.

    Dark streaks may indicate the presence of blood from higher up the digestive tract. Bleeding from the rectum produces recognizable blood. The former is more serious, as it may indicate polyps, colitis, or cancer. "Give Chaga tea," says Margi. "If it doesn't go away quickly, refer to a doctor."

    Gray, clay-like stool indicates a lack of bile and points to the gallbladder. "If the complexion is sallow, slightly yellow, the indication is weakness of the gallbladder. Use Werewolf root *Apocynum androsaemifolium*. If the complexion is jaundiced and more strongly yellow, the indication is blockage of the bile ducts; bile is entering the blood stream and not the stool. Remove congestion and heat from the gallbladder with Celandine *Chelidonium*, Red Root *Ceanothus*, Barberry root *Berberis vulgaris*, etc."

    Greenish discharges are usually dependent on an increase of acidity in the intestinal canal, with irritation and indigestion. It may in part be dependent upon the coloring matter of bile, which is thrown off by the feces in consequence of such irritation ascending the biliary duct (*Scudder*).

Shape

Stools that are too hard tend to come out in hard balls that are difficult to pass. These are called scybala. This indicates a lack of water and fiber, poor tone of the intestine, extended transit time, or difficulty in digesting food. Stools that are thin and long indicate too rapid transit time and poor assimilation.

Odor

The natural odor is evidence of normal activity throughout the entire tract. Diminution of odor is an indication of decreased functional activity; an increase indicates decomposition, bloating, gas, and inflammation. Foul scents: look to low stomach acid.

Substances

In severe diseases the stool will carry away tissue or substances from the body. The stool of tubercular patients is sometimes found to contain fat. Sugar occasionally appears in the excrement of diabetics. Blood in the stool arising from the small intestine will color the stool black, chocolate-brown or tarry black. These may also be dark streaks. Blood may also cause watery green excrement, as is observed occasionally in typhus. Mucus indicates inflammation of the walls of the colon (colitis). Epithelial cells, the lining of the intestines, are found in cholera.

Ease of passage

If the stool comes out easily and is easily completed, this indicates good tone in the rectum and sphincter.

If the stool comes out part way then recedes, or only partly comes away, or there is urging without stool, this indicates spasm interfering with peristalsis. Colicky pains, and alternating diarrhea and constipation often accompany this. This indicates irritable bowel syndrome, not constipation proper, which comes from a lack of tone. This should never be addressed with laxatives or purgatives, but with antispasmodics—Nux Vomica, Lobelia, Angelica.

If the stool is relatively well formed but does not come out easily or feels partly retained, this indicates good intestinal tone but poor rectal sphincter tone—Yellow Dock *Rumex crispus*, Lady's Mantle *Alchemilla vulgaris*, White Oak bark *Quercus alba*.

If the stool is dark and concentrated, this indicates true constipation. Strong laxatives should not be the first line of attack. Flax seed, freshly ground, or soaked overnight adding fruit and pineapple (with all its good digestive enzymes) are a good start on the problem. Fruit or prune juice with water may be added to lubricate the stool.

One easy recipe is 1 cup Oat bran, 1 cup Applesauce, half-cup Prune juice. Refrigerate covered.
Consume 2 tablespoons daily followed by a glass of warm water.

Oily foods such as Burdock root encourage the gallbladder to secrete more bile and lubricate the stool in this way. Psyllium seed adds fiber to stimulate peristalsis. Some people have an allergic reaction—do they get gas and bloating afterward? Try Chia seeds soaked overnight or in raw crackers.

Laxatives should be indicated by symptoms more than just "constipation." If symptoms include inactivity of the canal, straining at the stool, yet soft movement, with complexion yellow and red, try *Rumex crispus* (Yellow Dock root), *Juglans cinerea* or *J. nigra* (Butternut, Black Walnut). If there is closure of the gall ducts with poor lubrication of the bowels, try *Rheum palmatum* (Rhubarb root).

Bitters may be necessary to increase secretions from the intestinal wall: *Arctium lappa* (Burdock root) or *Berberis aquifolium* (Oregon Grape root).

Constipation or diarrhea while on a trip is often due to mild autonomic nervousness ("Where's the next bathroom? I don't like these strange places," etc.). "Here, Sweet leaf *Monarda fistulosa* may prove positive," says Matthew.

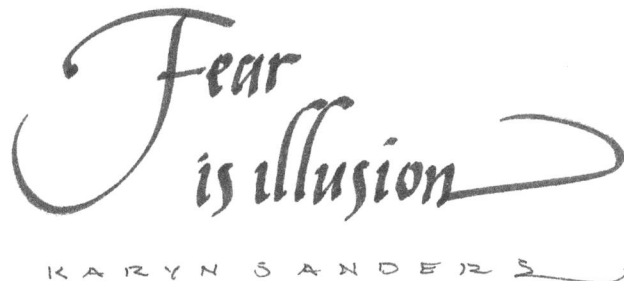

Fear is illusion

KARYN SANDERS

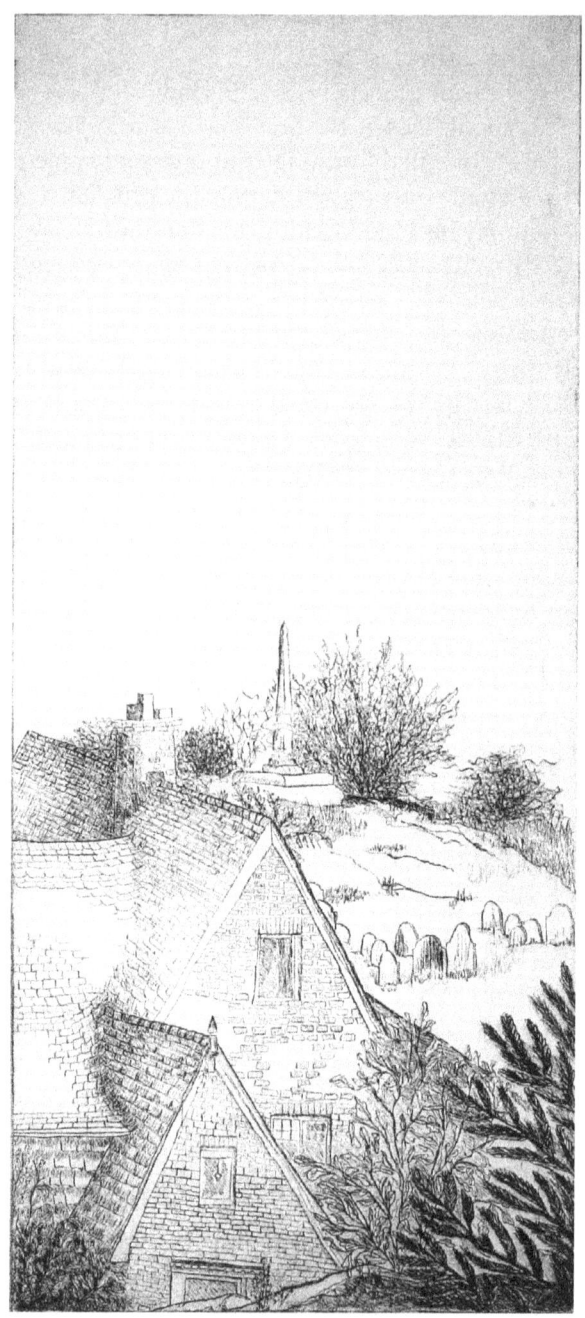

Old burial hill

CHAPTER 20

Stool indicators

General

The following table summarizes conditions that can be indicated through general stool analysis:

Stool indicator	Association
Slow transit time	Difficult-to-digest meals, poor digestive secretion, poor tone of the intestinal walls, and weak peristalsis
Rapid transit time	Easily digested food, watery food, non-absorption of water from the stool, closed pores of the intestine
Starts out hard and ends up loose	An untoned, unexercised colon and need for fiber
Diarrhea upon rising in morning	*Rumex crispus* (Yellow Dock)
Delay of stool upon rising	Slow transit time

(*Continued*)

(Continued)

Stool indicator	Association
Stool comes out part way then recedes	Spasm interfering with peristalsis; often with colicky pains, alternating diarrhea and constipation. Irritable bowel syndrome, not constipation. Antispasmodics
Stool is well-formed but does not come out easily	Good intestinal tone but poor rectal sphincter tone
Dry, hard, difficult, long transit time, dark.	True constipation
Loose, diarrhea	Weak, small intestine/spleen (Gentian, Bayberry), infections, worms, emotional—irritable bowel and absorption issues
Bloody diarrhea	Ischemic colitis (Comfrey, Cranesbill, Goldenseal, Marshmallow, Fenugreek)
Dry/hard/thin	Excess heat, contracted colon (Psyllium, Slippery Elm, Rhubarb)
Hard balls all stuck together	Constipation. Drink water, ½ body weight in ounces unless Kapha, add fruit and fiber, and Flax seeds, freshly ground
Narrow, noodle-like feces	Internalized tension, Crohn's disease, fibroids, tumors

Color

The following table summarizes conditions that can be indicated by stool color:

Stool color	Association
Green	Bile or chlorophyll
Red	Blood or beets, aspirin, red meat, or has increased intake of Vitamin C
Bright red	Rectum
Dark red	Stomach ulcer
Bloody diarrhea	Ulcerative colitis
Yellow	Liver fire (Rhubarb, Yellow Dock)

(*Continued*)

STOOL INDICATORS 201

(Continued)

Stool color	Association
Black	Blood or iron/magnesium. See the doctor
Yellow/white clay colored	Liver or gallbladder (Kelp, Oregon Grape root).
	Clay color—deficiency. Yellow—excess.
White clay	Gallbladder deficiency (Celandine tincture, one drop, twice a week, in water)
White greasy	Celiac disease, a response to gluten

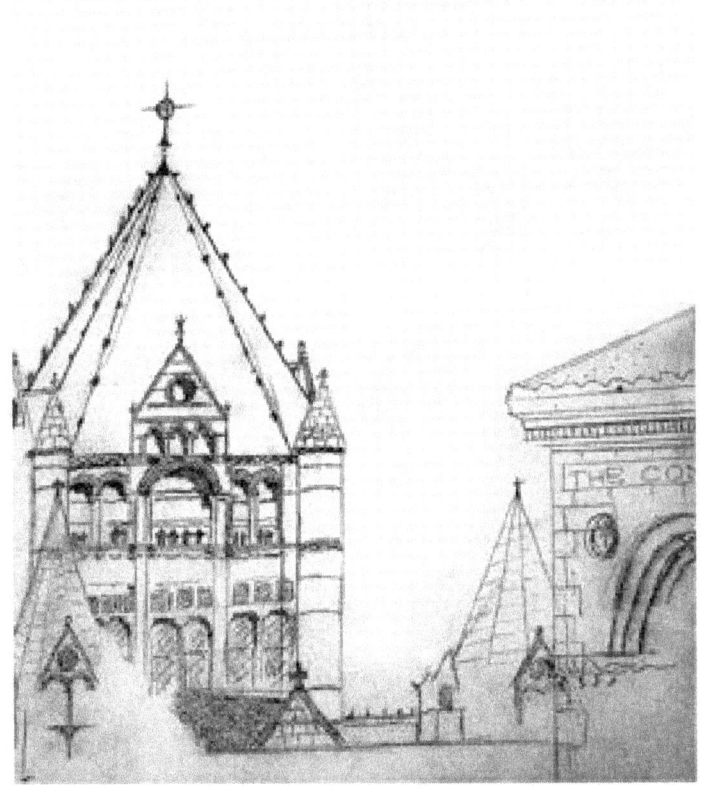

Working proof of Trinity Church Boston

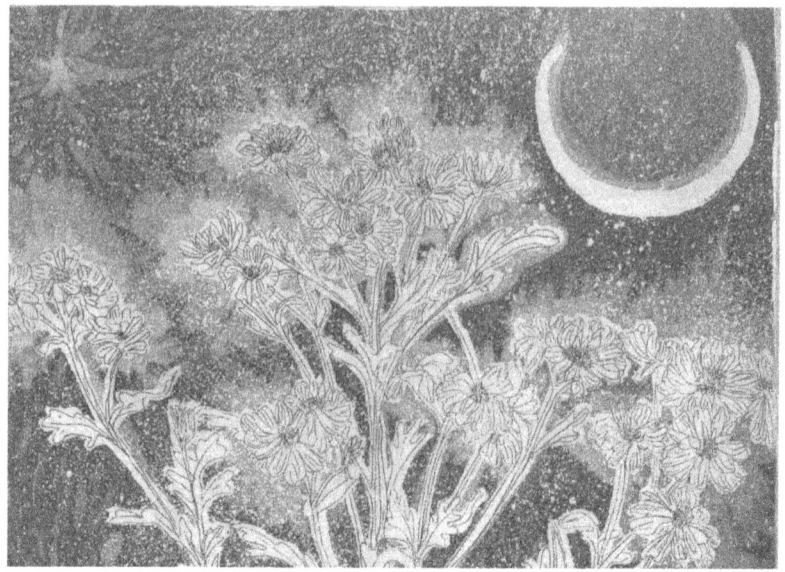
Segment of feverfew

CHAPTER 21

Urine analysis

Healthy urine is pale yellow with a steady stream. Easily begins and ends.

Have your client save the beginning stream of urine in a clean, clear glass, and the end stream in a separate clean, clear glass. In general, the following guidelines for appearance apply:

- Cloudy indicates infection
- Blood indicates irritation or a tumor
- Crystals indicate uric acid or calcium oxalate.

In addition, characteristics can have different associations, depending on whether they were in the first or last stream. The following table shows these associations:

If in first stream...	If in last stream...
Blood in the bladder	Blood in the kidney
Clean and healthy	No blood, not kidney

(Continued)

(Continued)

If in first stream…	If in last stream…
Cloudy indicates infection in bladder	Cloudy indicates infection in kidney
Lack of foam in stream	"Low hormones." M.W.

Urine color

The following table summarizes conditions that can be indicated by urine color:

Color	Association
Clear	Yin. Cold. (Cranberry). Too much water
Dark yellow/orange	Yang. Hot. Spleen, pancreas (Cornsilk, Red Root, Agrimony). Too little water. Pregnancy. B vitamin use
Cloudy/milky	Excess protein or infection (Gravel Root, Buchu)
Red	Blood (Collinsonia, Agrimony, Sweet Birch)

Urine smell

The following table summarizes conditions that can be indicated by urine smell:

Smell	Association
Foul	Infection (Agrimony, Sweet Birch)
Sweet	Too much glucose, ketones. Look to diabetes. "Smells like cotton candy."

Urine texture

The following table summarizes conditions that can be indicated by foam in toilet:

Symptom	Association
Foam in urine	Full bladder, strong stream
Foam, swollen legs and eyes	See doctor
Bubbles remain after flushing	Could be albumin, protein; look to kidney disease, lupus, diabetes

CHAPTER 22

Drop-pulse testing

*S*ections in italics are from *The Practicing Herbalist IV* and are copyrighted.

Learn to relax your mind and gain confidence with Drop-Pulse Testing. Clients love this testing, for they are directly involved in the process. A great way to narrow down the herbal choices and find the ones most suited to the individual.

Test tinctures, dried herbs, or fresh herbs to sense responses. Your client is joining their energies with the herbs to sense a response.

I have studied pulse with many teachers over these past decades. The information was daunting and unapproachable. When I sat at the knee of Matthew Wood the light dawned. Then William Morris giggled himself into my life. William's book honoring his mentor Li Shi-Zhen's Pulse Studies, an illustrated guide I highly recommend. Next, find where he teaches and sit at his knee! Experiencing the pulse with the teacher present is invaluable. I asked herb sister Kay Parent to share her thoughts on knowing the pulse.

The experience of pulse

"To approach the inner wrist, to hold the hands, to feel the temperature and texture of the skin is to enter an inner world where the body and spirit start to speak in an immediate way about the past and present. Asking permission to touch is the overture. Then holding both hands calms the body and encourages deeper questions or observation to rise to the surface. Approaching by first looking at the color of the nails, inner coloring of the palm noting how the hands functions in their daily life. Engaging the client lightly while your ears widen to start listening deeper.

Approaching lung (right), heart (left), feeling both at the same time, getting a sense of the seat of blood and oxygen, the first burner. The same then with liver (left), stomach (right), a sense of how all is received into the body and cleared in the second burner. Finally, kidney (left) and Thyroid/Endocrine (right), where lower back speaks and body gives a sense of how all the systems are working together.

Of special interest is always the back body, the spine, the nerves that feed the organs and the flow of cerebral spinal fluid. The pulses have a voice of their own. They speak of the physical body, the energetic body and sometimes the light touch of finger to pulse will bring up a question which is neither physical or energetic, but pertinent to the person's tender understanding of where they are in life.

My usual manner is to look at the tongue first with the client; to gaze upon it has a humor about it that is disarming to both client and practitioner. Then we approach the face and finally the pulse. I find the pulses the most intimate and I intrude on them with a slow, deliberate cadence showing respect for their boundaries. Most times the organs through the pulses convey their wisdom easily and are delighted to be heard, but if they are silent and deep and don't wish to speak, we stop and honor the reticence and silence.

Using Matthew Wood's pulse testing for herbs offers client, practitioner and herb an adventurous, collaborative way of working together. It allows the herbs to speak directly with the body and verify or negate what we have intuited or thought. A humbling moment!

All in all, my journey with pulses is the privilege of hearing the whisperings of the spirit and the nudging of the body."

Kay Parent, herbalist/mentor, AHG

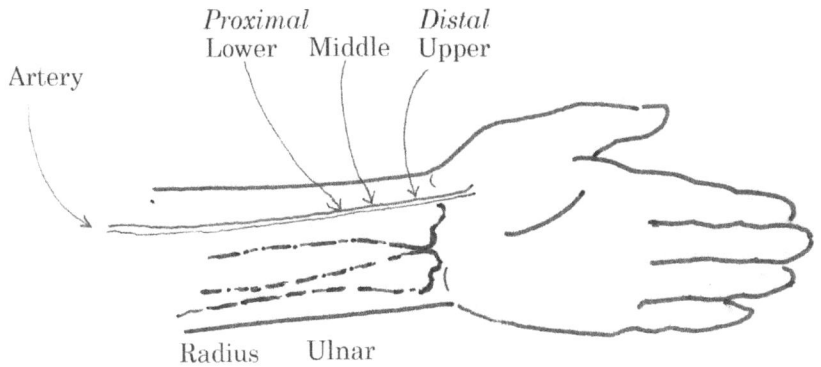

Pulse position correspondences

Family history		Person now	
Left wrist		**Right wrist**	
Surface	Deep	Surface	Deep
Small intestine	Heart	Large intestines	Lung
Gallbladder	Liver	Stomach	Spleen
Bladder	Kidneys	Kidney Yang	Pericardium
			Triple heater
More simply:			
Heart		Lungs	
Liver		Stomach	
Kidney water		Kidney Fire	
Weak = inherited constitution, essence, must rest		Weak = Acquired constitution, vitality, diet, exercise	

Which fingertip is hit first?
Are the pulses even on both wrists?

In Chinese medicine the Pericardium is the outer protective shield of the heart. The Triple Heater is the functional relationship between organs that regulate water. Kidney water is the endocrine system in active fiery manifestation. Heart stores the spirit Shen. Liver stores, and is in charge of spreading Chi. Kidneys store the essence. Lungs, pneuma, is the spirit from birth to death. Yin Organs are the heart, lungs, spleen, liver, and kidneys. The pericardium's function is to produce, transform regulate & store Chi, blood, Jing, Shen and fluids. Yang Organs are the gallbladder, stomach, small intestine, large intestine, bladder and triple burner. Yang Organs receive, break down, and absorb that part of the food, which will be transformed into fundamental substances, and transport and excrete the unused portion.

Hold the elbow with your hand, cradling the relaxed arm of the person in the crook of your arm. Keep a breath between fingers holding the pulse points. The ultra-basics are to look at tubes, pumps, fluids and ground substance. The ideal pulse has root, runs from side to side beneath fingers deep, has stomach Chi, has Shen: stability of rate, amplitude and is evenly distributed between positions. When the pulse is weak build the essence. When the pulse changes, is weak, feeble or absent supplement the essence. When forceful eliminate and purge. When the pulse has tension, is wiry and tense like a guitar string, treat the nervous system. When nothing is there the interstitial tissue is wet "cotton" between the skin and surface of the vessel. When nothing is there look to hypothyroid, lack of movement, depression. When it is ropey it indicates atherosclerosis.

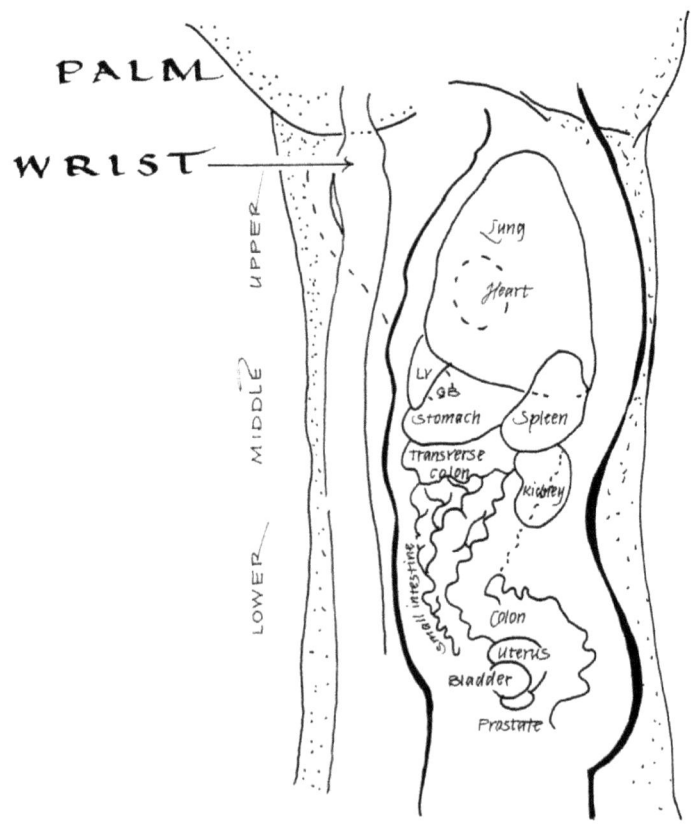

When holding your own wrist up, the body is reflected from the lungs to reproductive organs.

First ask permission to touch the body. Feel the palm and softly stroke up the inner arm. Compare palm to arm.

The pointer finger is first toward the thumb on the radial side.

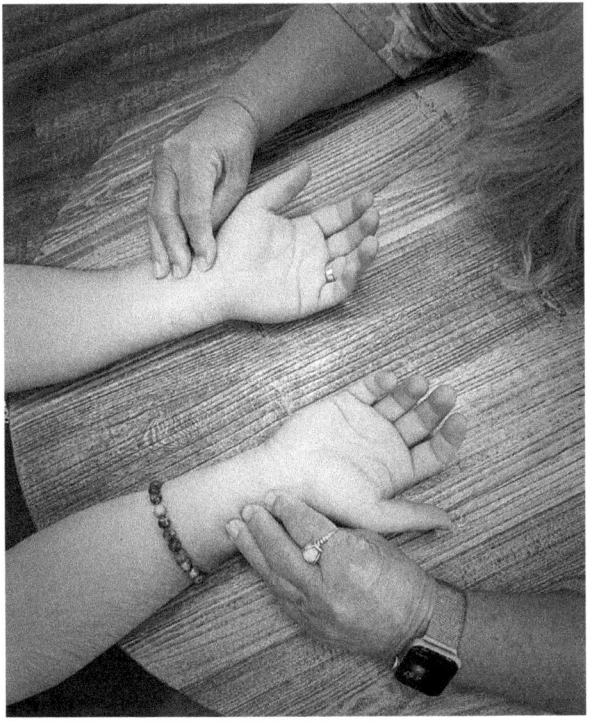

Sit holding the wrist with fingertips in the gully between tendons on the radial side. Keep the finger tips a breath apart. Some are more comfortable simply laying the pointer, fire and ring fingers in the gully. Note pulses on both wrists.

Have your tinctures or herbs lined up.

Open the bottle a comfortable distance from the client. (The herbs begin working as soon as the scent reaches the olfactory bulb.)

Do not allow the dropper to touch the skin.

Apply a drop of tincture and swipe horizontally across the wrist. Each application in a new area. Do not allow the name of the herb to be read.

Observe the changes in the pulse. Observers watch: Eyes, pupils, skin color, shoulders, breath, tears, laughter.

Ask the client for their perceptions before offering yours.

You can record your observations and compare the next time they are seen. One herb will speak clearly to you!

This is a simple way to choose between herbs. Have fun.

CHAPTER 23

Quicksight confirmations

Use these pages as a "Monarch note" version of all that has been shared before. For quick reference, two pages will contain visual and written reminders for each organ or body part. Remember to note the body type: Vata, Pitta or Kapha.

General indications

Hot indicates upward motion	↑ Red	Fast
Cold indicates downward motion	↓ Pale	Slow
Damp indicates inward stagnation	Puffy ~~~	Mucus—heavy sing-song voice
Dry indicates outward evaporation	Insomnia	Dark Itchy urine
Wind indicates uncontrolled movement	~~~ Irregularities	
Concave areas indicate	Prolapse, atonic conditions	
Convex areas indicates	Weak tissue Wet	Boggy stagnation

Skin with tight, dense, clear porosity indicates a strong constitution. Large-pored skin indicates a more sensitive, "open to receive" constitution.

Pathology may exist when one side is different.

> "Liver rules the smooth flow of emotions across the body, then stomach, then bowels." W.Le.

Color

White	Pale Anemic	Shock	Lung
Gray	Large intestine		
Ruddy	Gallbladder		
Red	Heat Heart		
Yellow	Gallbladder		
Yellow/brown	Deficiency in stomach		
Lemon yellow	Pancreas		
Blue	Lack of oxygen		
Purple	Indicates infection, stagnation		
Black	Chemotherapy, extreme fungal infection		

Pupils

Shen, spirit, presence, who is home? "Pupils should be even, round and accommodating." W.Le.

Alternating—adrenal stress. Dilated—lack of enervation from low blood sugar.

QUICKSIGHT CONFIRMATIONS 213

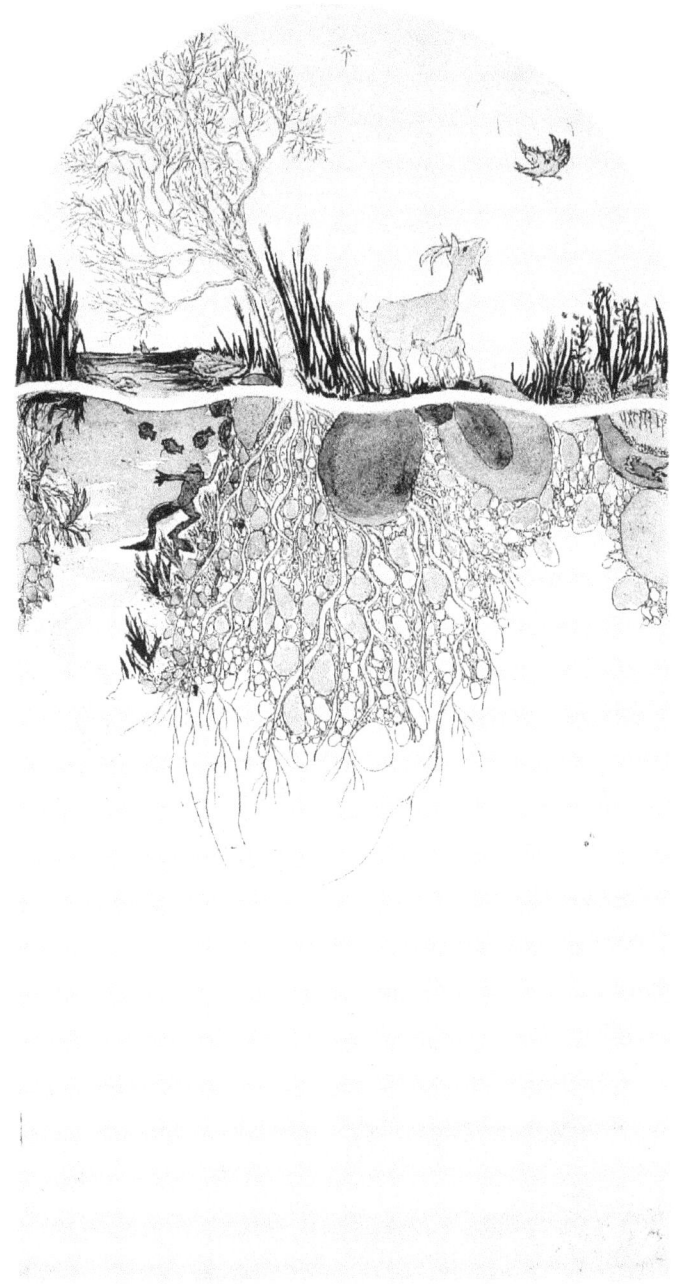

I'll drink to that

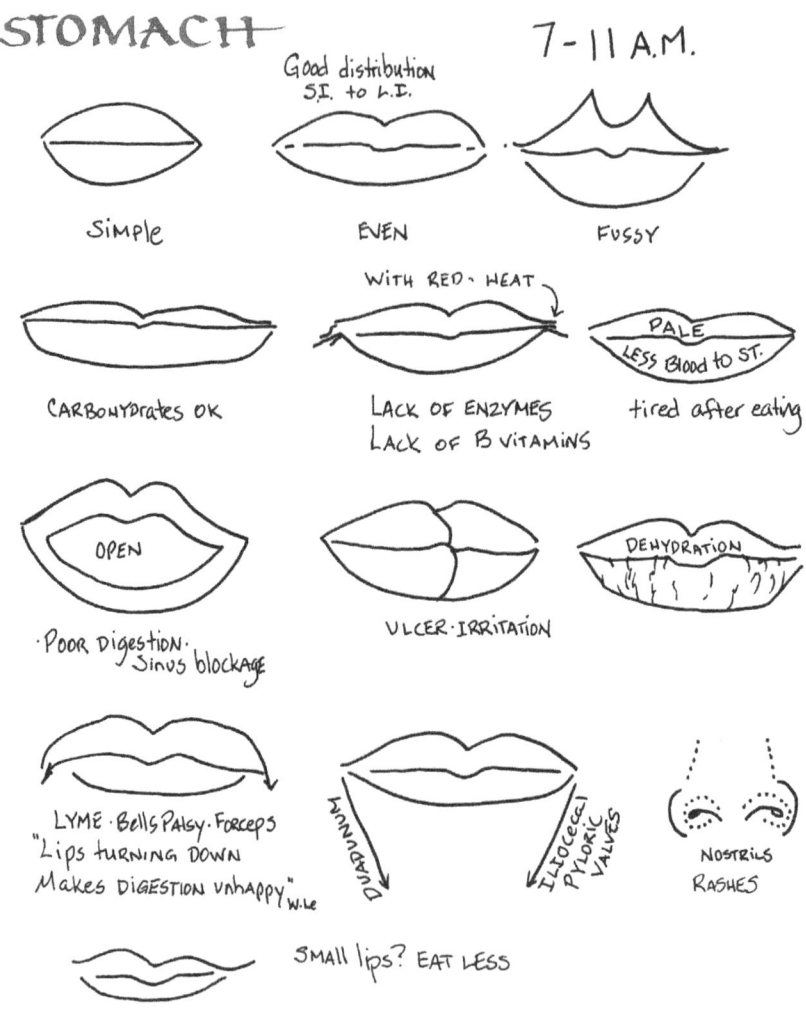

"Charity begins at home, Begin with the stomach" William LeS.

Await indications of three

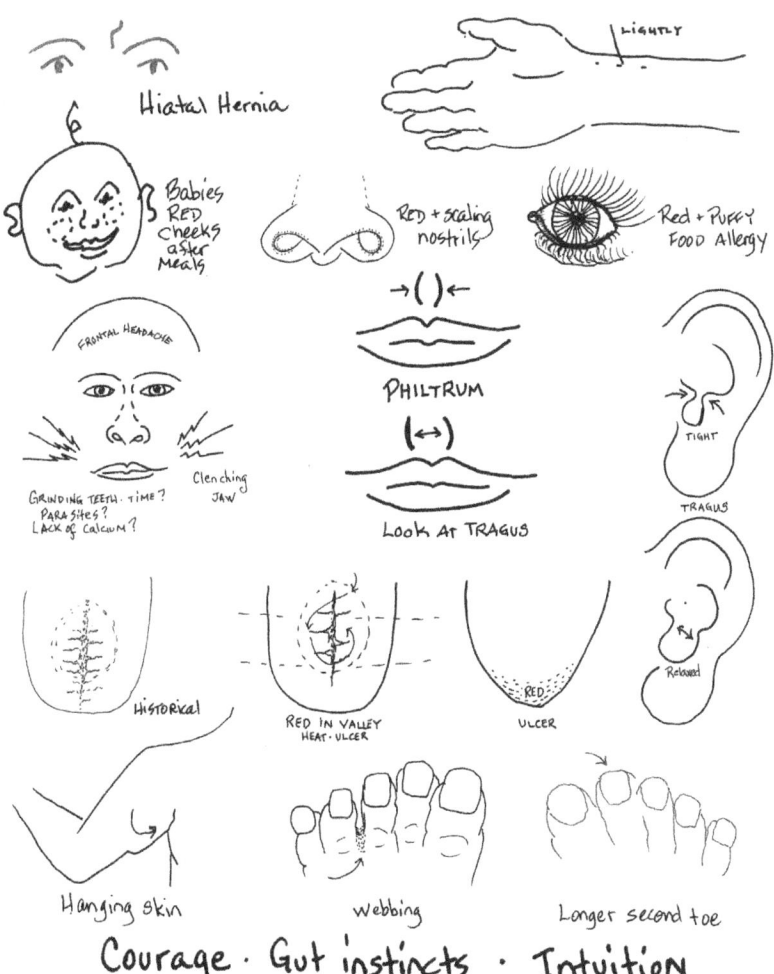

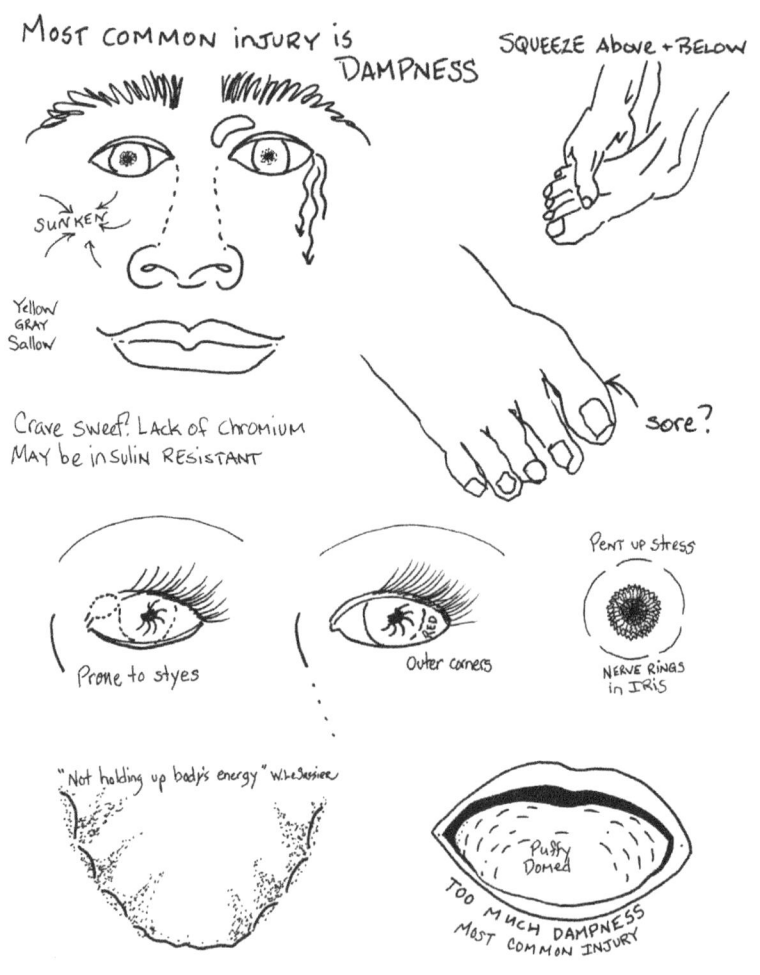

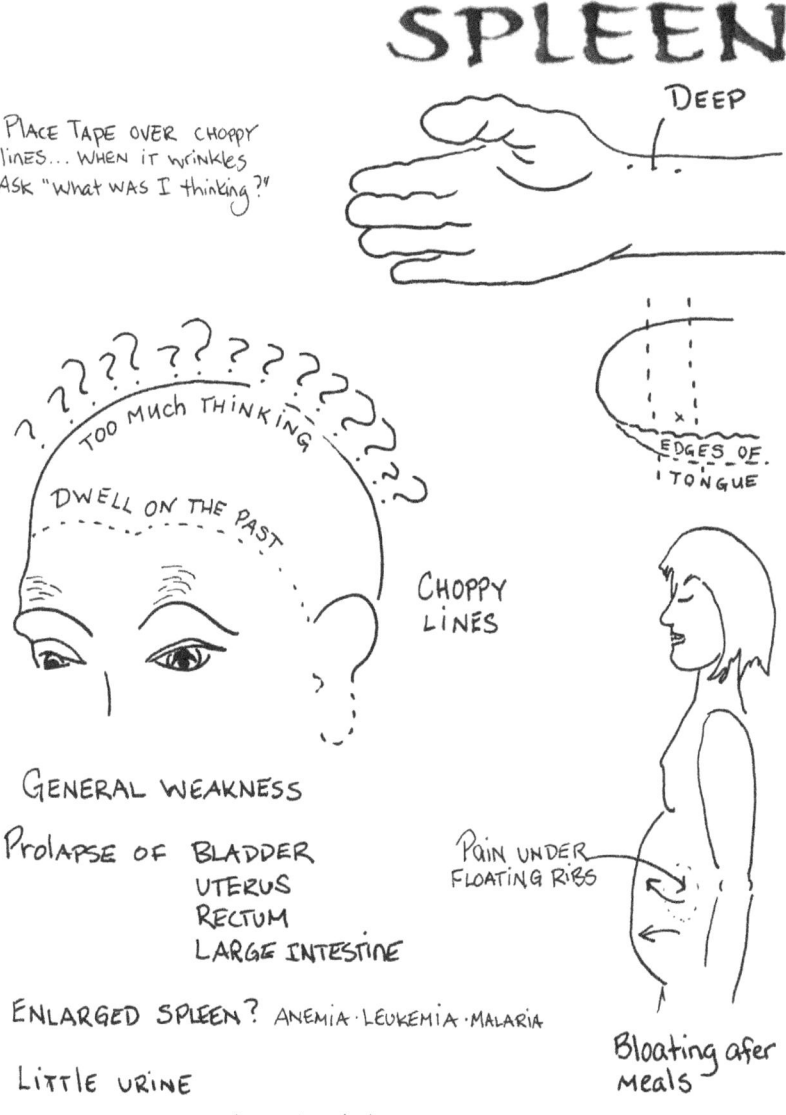

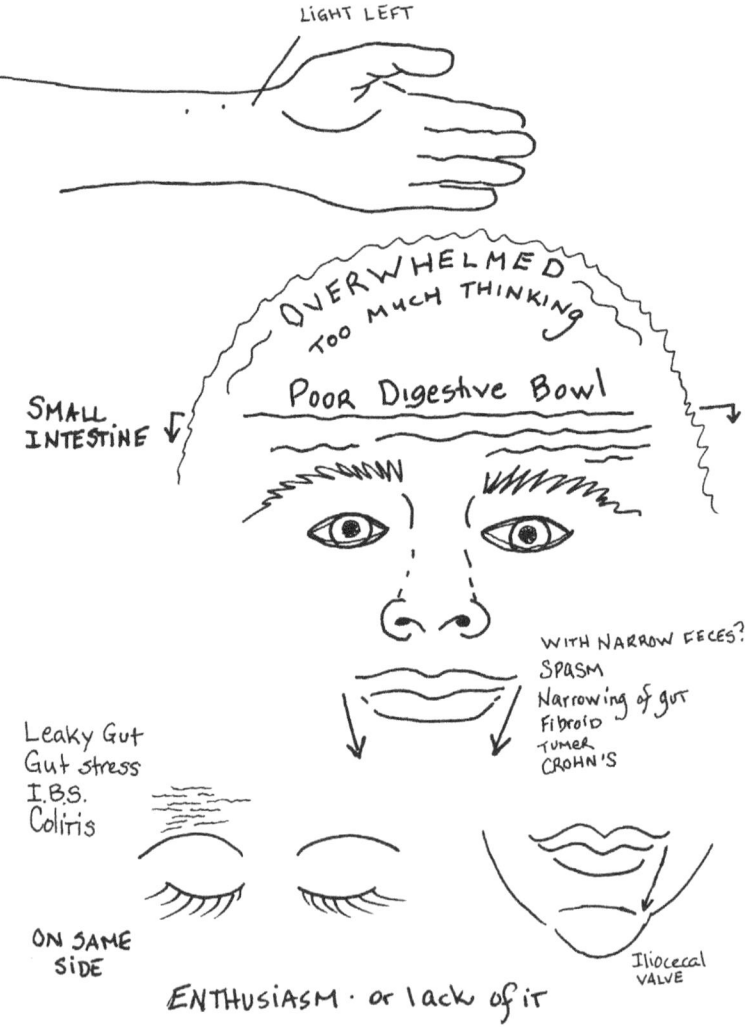

SMALL INTESTINE

1½ HOURS AFTER EATING feel tired

1-3 P.M. TIRED

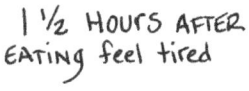
SMALL Scaling Red Pimples = FOOD REACTION

AVOID: spicy
sweet
coffee
citrus
ginger

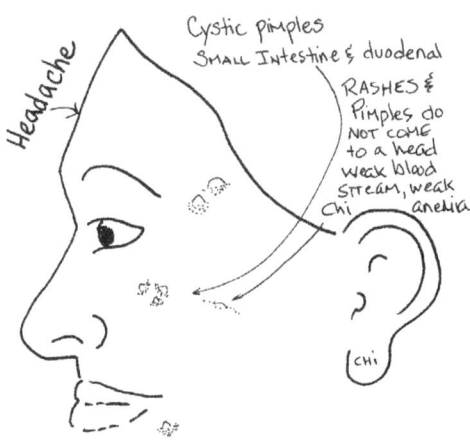

Headache

Cystic pimples
Small Intestine & duodenal
RASHES & Pimples do NOT COME to a head
weak blood stream, weak Chi
anemia
(chi)

Porocity of Membranes

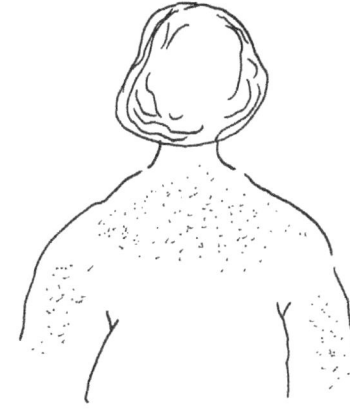

The effective intake of NUTRITION

LOW STOMACH ACID
& lack of calcium + iron

SHEETS of pimples
Cold trapped under the surface
LACK of Vit C, Zinc, Selenium?

← LACK OF EFA's

EXCESS EXCITEMENT

Await indications of three

LARGE INTESTINE

AWAKEN 5-7 A.M.

T·E·N·S·I·O·N

Gray Cheeks

Food Allergies

Blackheads in creases. What color is in the crease?

Anywhere on body → SKIN TAGS = TOXICITY OF AREA BELOW
L.I + Lymphatics undigested protein

SORE 3rd RIB in line with nipple

STRESS & TENSION
Feces white? colitis

Muscle Tension Headache

BACK THIRD

EMOTIONAL SECURITY
Releasing "Being in the flow"

OVER-ANXIOUS
HARD TIME LETTING GO

QUICKSIGHT CONFIRMATIONS 221

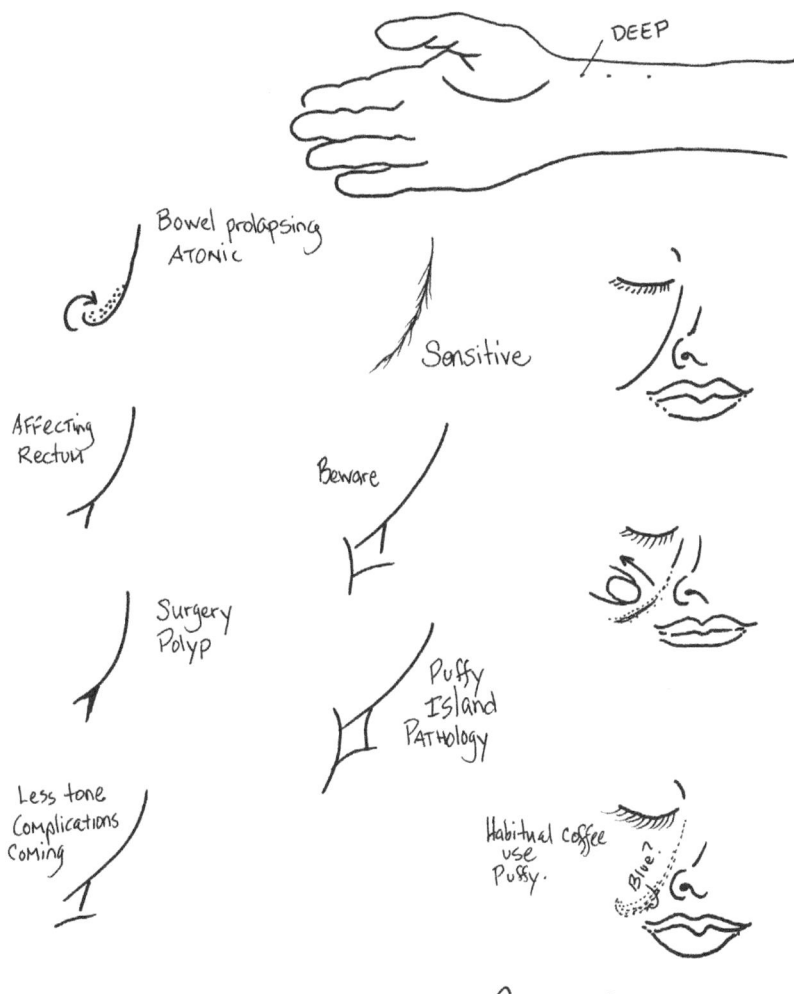

Await indications of three

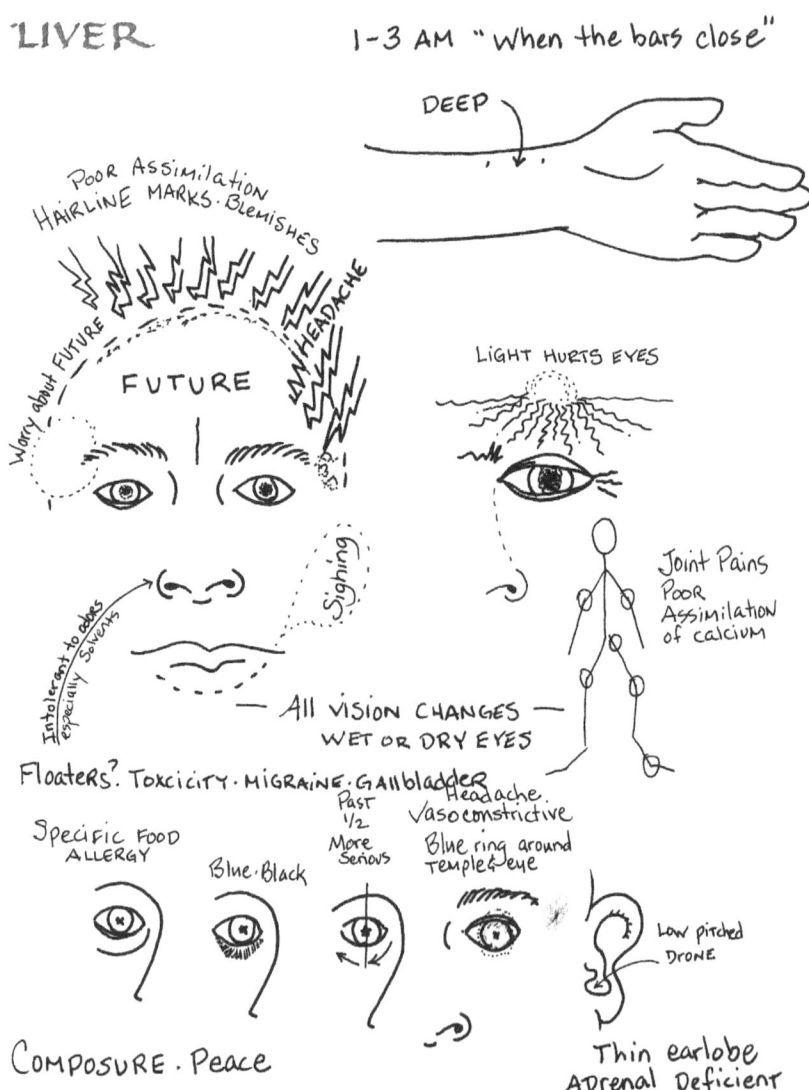

QUICKSIGHT CONFIRMATIONS

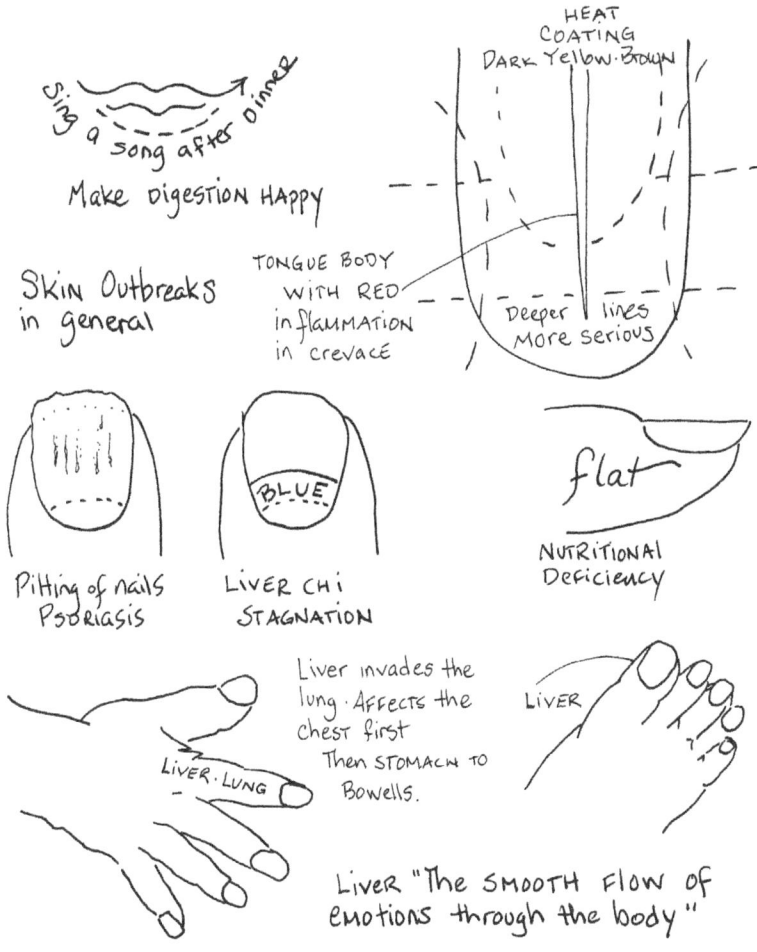

Await indications of three

GALLBLADDER

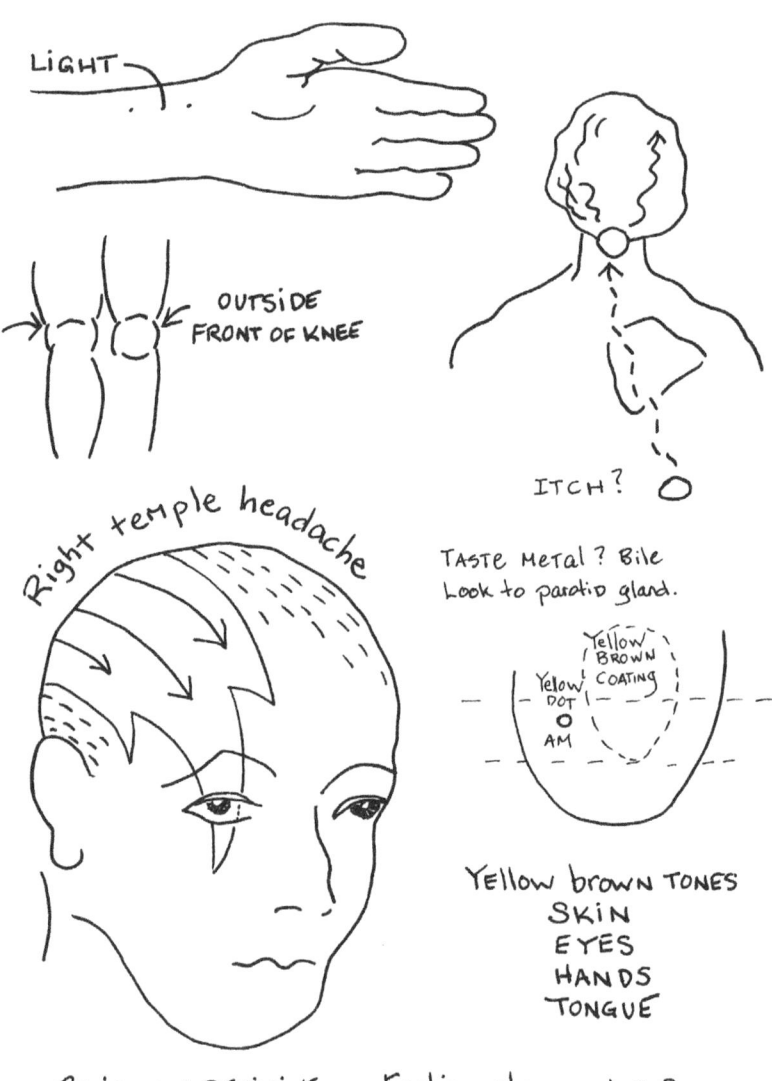

GALLBLADDER

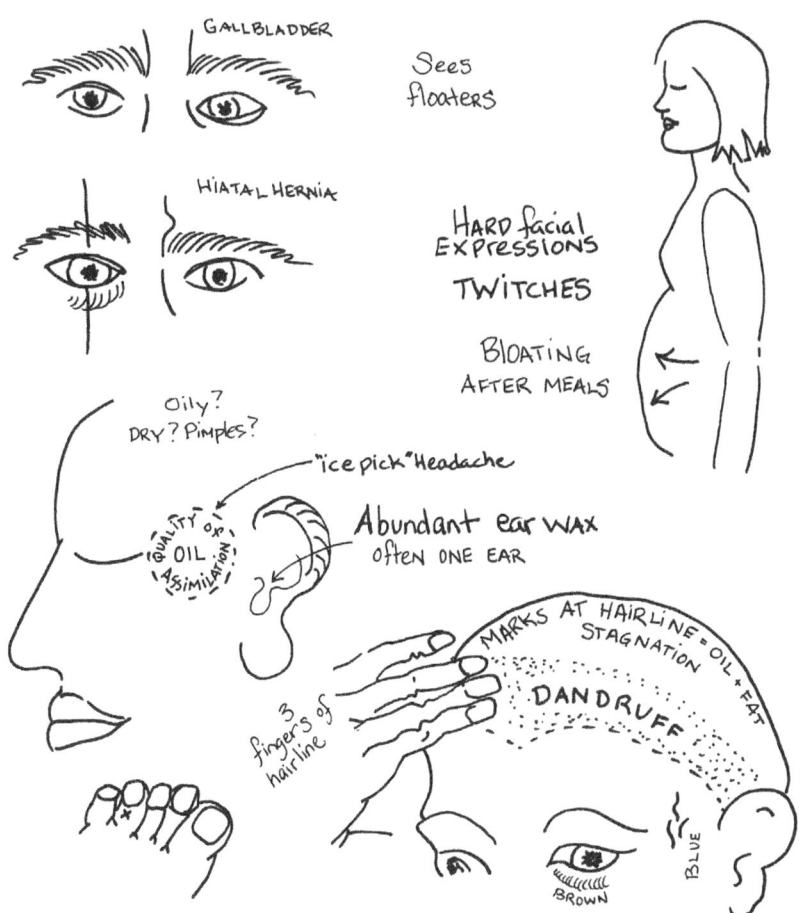

Boundary Issues   passive aggressive

Feeling Galled · Repressed burning anger · Indecision

Await indications of three

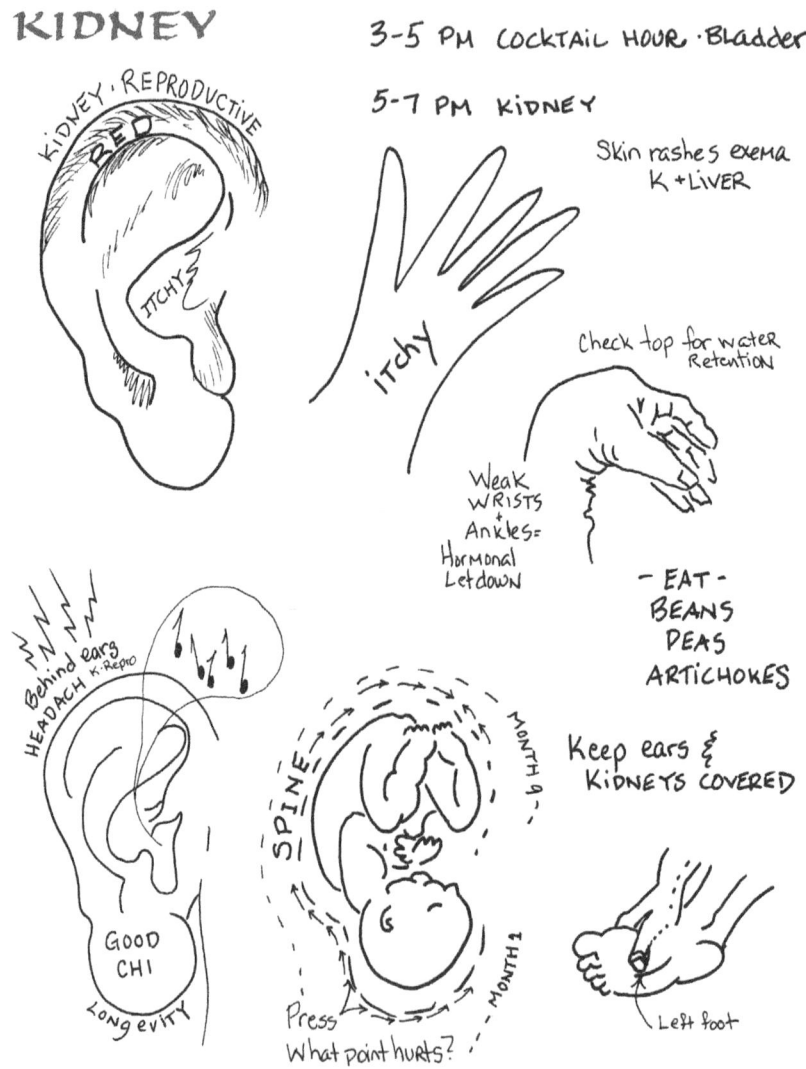

KIDNEY

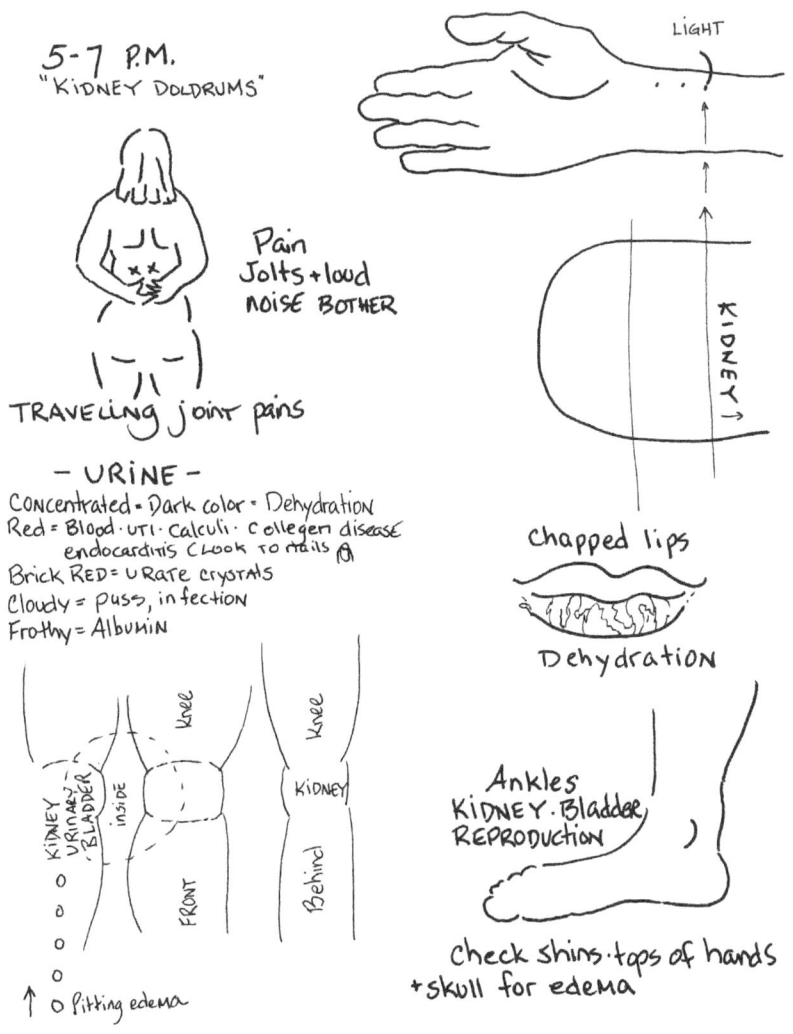

LUNG

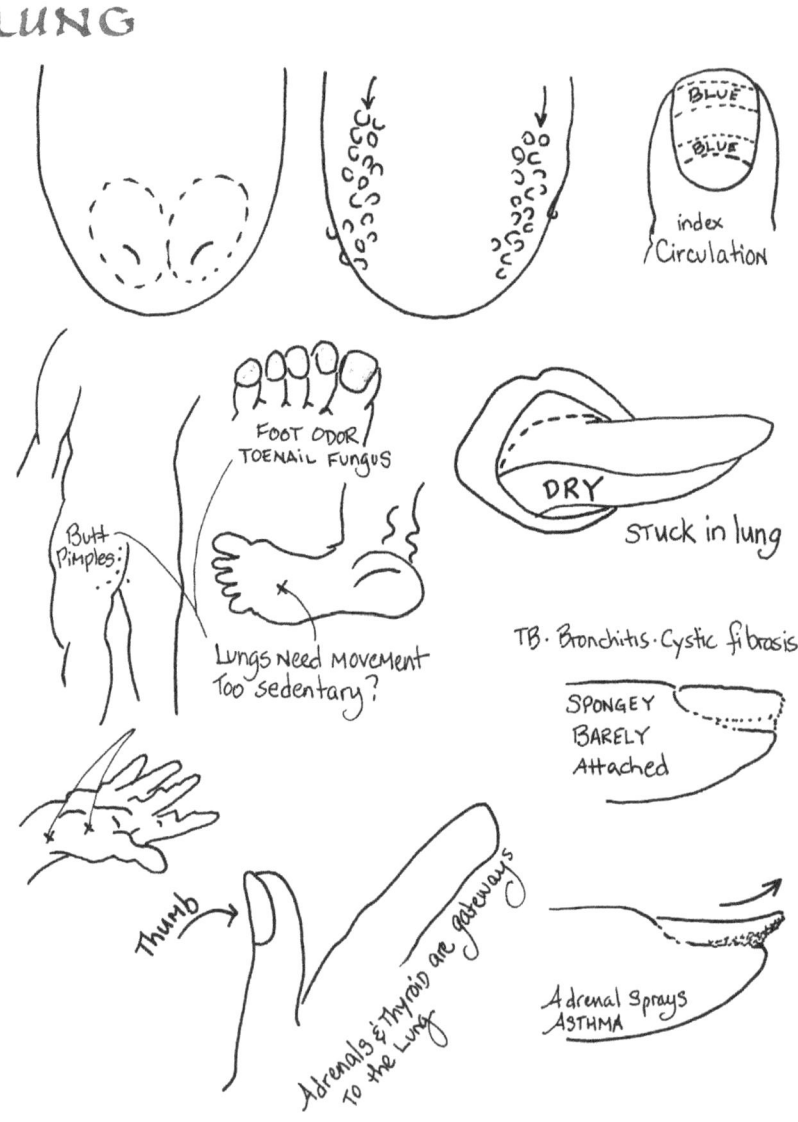

Await indications of three

QUICKSIGHT CONFIRMATIONS 229

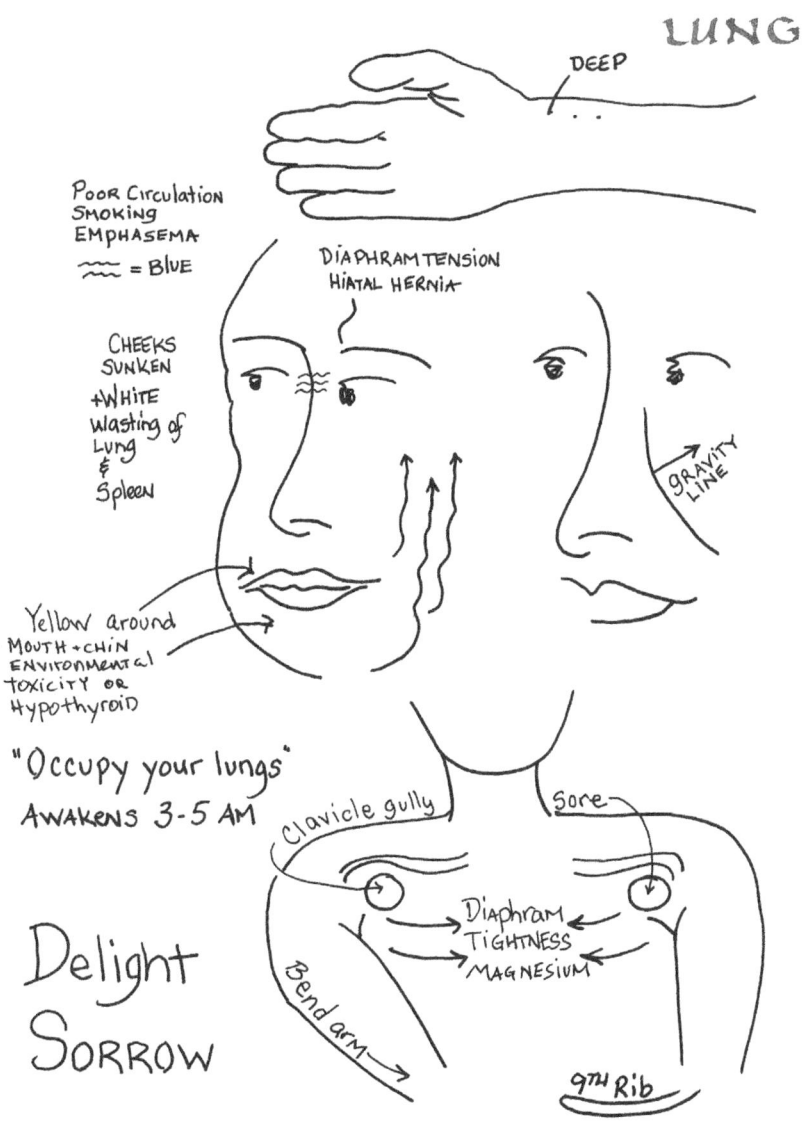

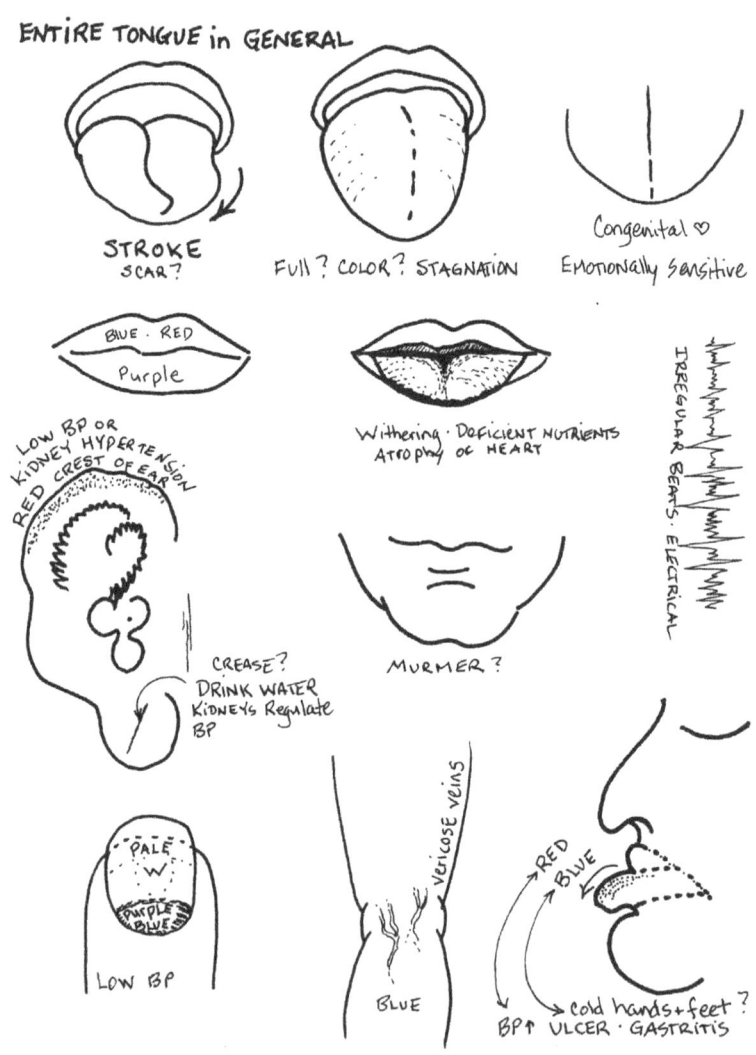

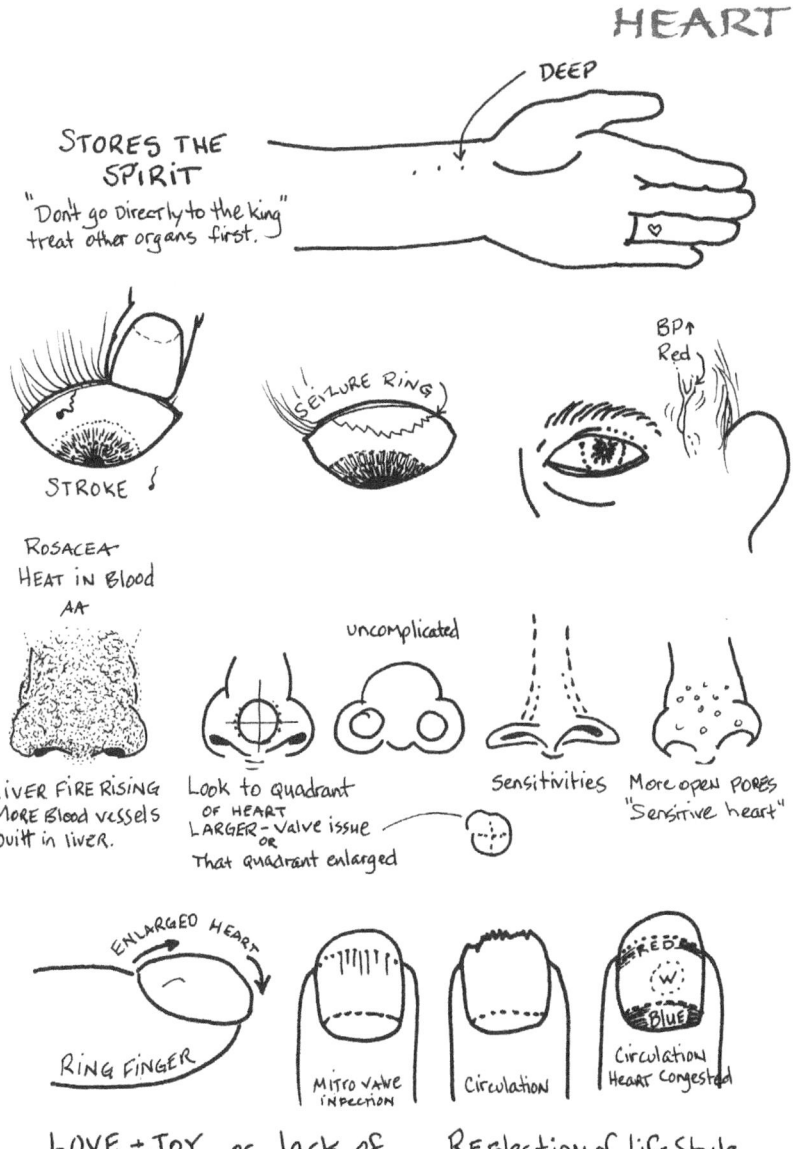

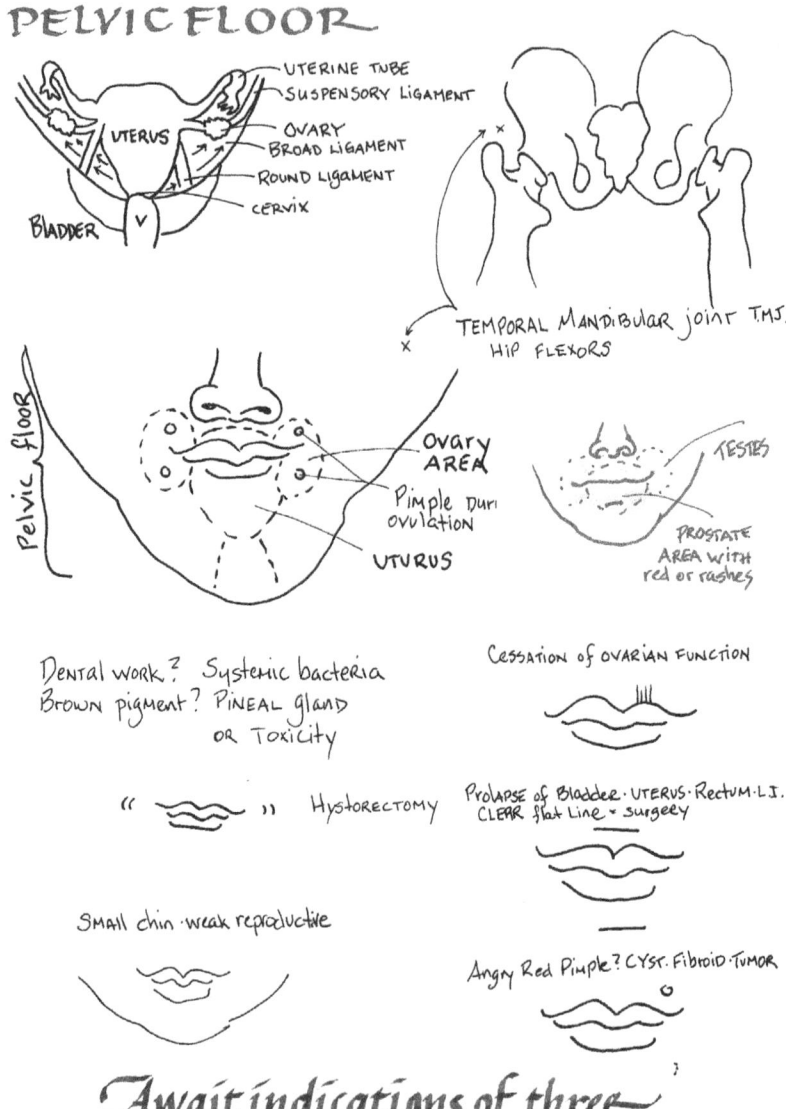

QUICKSIGHT CONFIRMATIONS 233

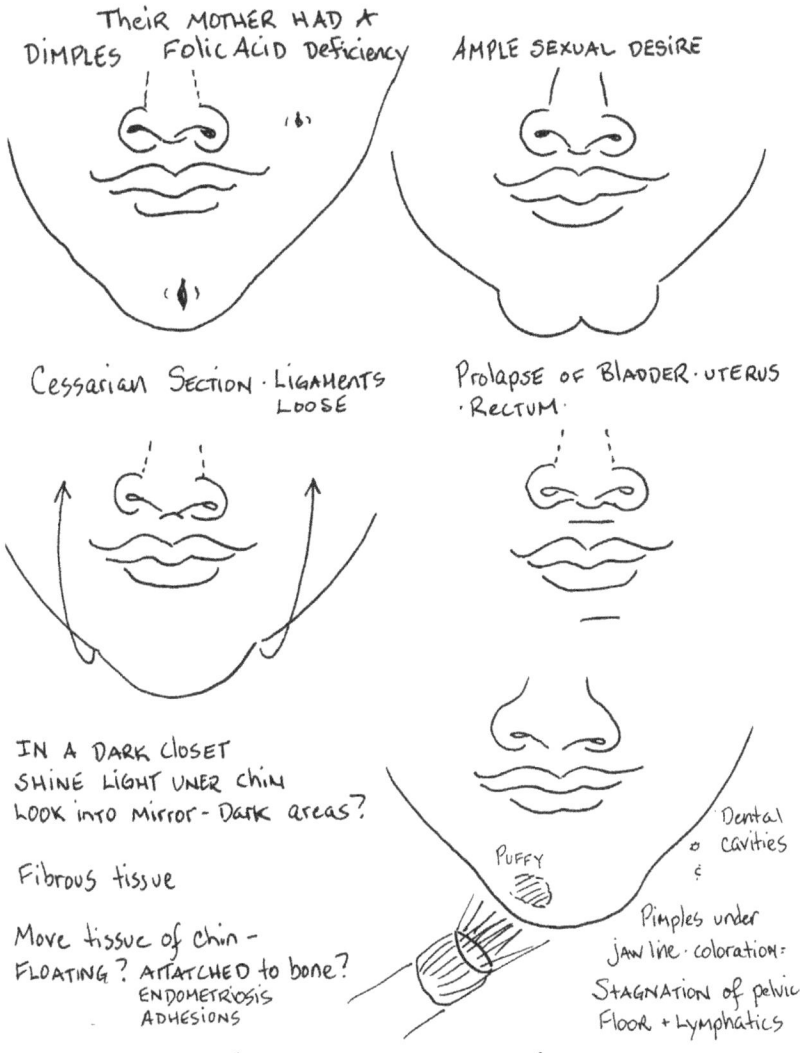

PELVIC FLOOR

DIMPLES — Their MOTHER HAD A FOLIC ACID DEFICIENCY

AMPLE SEXUAL DESIRE

Cessarian SECTION · LIGAMENTS LOOSE

Prolapse OF BLADDER · UTERUS · RECTUM ·

IN A DARK CLOSET
SHINE LIGHT UNER CHIN
LOOK INTO MIRROR - DARK areas?

Fibrous tissue

Move tissue of chin —
FLOATING? ATTACHED to bone?
ENDOMETRIOSIS
ADHESIONS

PUFFY

Dental cavities

Pimples under jaw line · coloration =
STAGNATION of pelvic
Floor + Lymphatics

EMOTIONAL · SEXUAL · HISTORY

APPENDIX

Table of contents to The Practicing Herbalist meeting with clients – reading the body IV

The full edition is 563 pages hardbound. I share recipes, formulations, observations, and stories as they came alive on the pages. It is my legacy and my love. With great respect for all of us learning how to practice well with open hearts and good boundaries. Invest in your tools. Take time for your own wellbeing, Margi.

Dedication
Acknowledgements
Foreword to the Fourth edition shared by Sajah Popham
The Beginning
    1. About Me
    2. Starting a Practice
    3. Seeing Clients
    4. Modern Marketing
    5. Accounting
    6. Book List
    7. Asking Questions
    8. Sample Blank Intake
    9. Sous Vide
    10. Calcium Deficiency

11. Human Papilloma Virus (HPV)
12. Living with Cancer
13. A Simplistic View of Individual Cancers
14. Mushrooms in Cancer Therapy
15. Preparing for Surgery and Scar Tissue
16. Experimental Protocols for Lyme Disease
17. David Winston AHG Tick-Borne Diseases
18. An Herbal Approach to Lyme and Possible Co-infections Kate Gilday
19. David Dalton—Lyme & Flower Essences
20. Lyme Disease Update Wendy Snow Fogg
21. Decreasing Antidepressant Use
22. Autoimmune Disease Insulin Resistance
23. Relieving Chronic Pain
24. Disrupted Sleep Patterns
25. Headaches and Head Trauma
26. Understanding the Endocrine Cascade
27. Understanding Intrinsic Factor
28. Covid Viral Infections
29. Vitamins, Minerals & Amino Acids
30. Voice
31. Assessing the Energetics of a Condition
32. Visual Observations
33. Constitutional Body Types
34. Examining Color
35. Organ/Body Correspondences
36. Examining the Face
37. Examining Ears
38. Examining the Eyes
39. Examining the Nose
40. Examining the Mouth and Teeth and Lips
41. Examining the Chin
42. Examining the Tongue
43. Specific Tongue Indications
44. The Hands
45. Examining the Fingernails
46. Large Intestine Lines
47. Elimination
48. Urine

APPENDIX 237

49. Pulses
50. Quicksight Confirmations
51. Planetary Responsibility
52. Resources
53. List of Artwork
54. Index of Kay Parent's Calligraphy
55. Common to Latin Names
56. Index

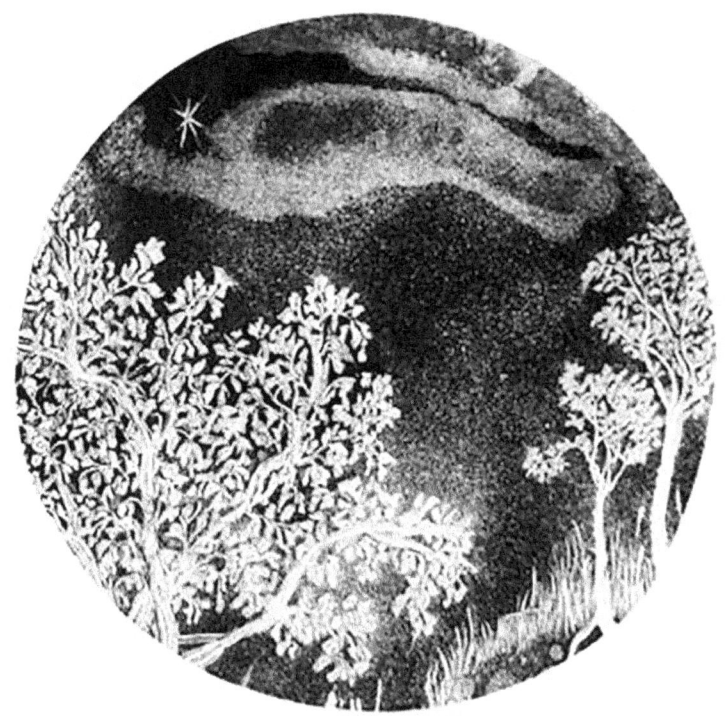

Wishing star

INDEX

ACTH. *See* adrenocorticotropic hormone
ADD. *See* attention deficit disorder
addictive behaviors, 76
adenomas, toxic, 99
ADH. *See* anti-diuretic hormone
adrenal glands, 81. *See also* endocrine cascade
   adrenal cortex, 82
   adrenal medulla, 82
   aldosterone, 82
   androgenic steroids, 82
   corticosterone, 82
   epinephrine, 83
   herbs for adrenals, 85
   hydrocortisone, 82
   indications for, 83–84
   norepinephrine, 83
   nutrition for, 84
   supplements for, 85
adrenaline. *See* epinephrine
adrenocorticotropic hormone (ACTH), 75. *See also* hypothalamus

air-filter/ionizer, 20
aldosterone, 82. *See also* adrenal glands
alpha cells, 102. *See also* pancreas
American Ginseng, 78, 85, 96
American Herbalists Guild, 14
amygdala, 68–69. *See also* pineal gland
amylin, 102. *See also* pancreas
androgenic steroids, 82. *See also* adrenal glands
anti-diuretic hormone (ADH), 81
Arnica flower, 77
attention deficit disorder (ADD), 76
Ayurvedic medicine, 43

B-12 rich foods, 77
beta cells, 102. *See also* pancreas
bile acids, 66
bladder, 131–132
body's communication network. *See* organ/body correspondences
body type indications, 211–212
Burdock root, 77

calcaneonavicular coalition, 70
calcium, 101
camp bed, 36
capsules, 20
cash sale, 29
Catnip personality, 20
Chamomile personality, 20
Chickweed, 85, 96
chin examination, 163–164
cholesterol, 66
client
    files, 35
    observation, 135–136
client intake, 45
    creating life timeline, 45–46
    men, 61–63
    sample of intake form, 46–54
    women, 54–61
Coleus, 96
color indications, 113
    black, 120–121
    blue, 119–120
    body, 212
    fingernail, 183–187
    gray, 118, 130
    green, 114–115, 132
    orange, 119
    purple, 121
    red, 115–117, 132
    stool, 195, 200–201
    white, 113–114
    yellow, 118–119
"compl e ment", 14
"compl i ment", 15
composting, 15–16
constitution of person, 136
consultation room and classroom, 36–39
corticosterone, 82. *See also* adrenal glands
corticotrophin releasing hormone (CRH), 75. *See also* hypothalamus
CRH. *See* corticotrophin releasing hormone
cruciferous vegetables, 99

Cryptococcus neoformans, 70
cycles of life, 66

delta cells, 102. *See also* pancreas
desk area, 23, 25–28
dimethyltryptamine (DMT), 69
DMT. *See* dimethyltryptamine
dopamine, 75. *See also* hypothalamus
dosha, 43
drop-pulse testing, 205
    experience of pulse, 206
    guide to herbal diagnosis, 207–210
    pulse position correspondences, 207
Drum, Ryan, 33

EarthSong Herbals, 11–12
EFAs. *See* essential fatty acids
electromagnetic field (EMF), 67
EMF. *See* electromagnetic field
endocrine cascade, 65
    adrenal glands, 81–85
    hormone, 66
    hyperparathyroid, 92
    hyperthyroid, 98–101
    hypothalamus, 72–78
    hypothyroid, 93–98
    ovaries, 106–110
    pancreas, 101–106
    parathyroid gland, 90–91
    pineal gland, 66–72
    pituitary gland, 78–81
    testes, 110–112
    thyroid gland, 86–90
endocrine system, 65
environmental consciousness and health, 14
epinephrine, 83. *See also* adrenal glands
essential fatty acids (EFAs), 101
esterone, 108. *See also* ovaries
estriol-DHEA, 107. *See also* ovaries
eye examination, 145, 147–150
    eyebrow examination, 143–144
    eye socket, 146
    general eye conditions, 145–146
eyelid, below, 153–154
eye socket, 146

facial analysis, 137–141
fingernail examination, 183
　color/conditions and indications, 183–187
Flint, Margi, 2–8
follicle stimulating hormone (FSH), 75, 79, 107. *See also* hypothalamus; ovaries; pituitary gland
formula preparation area, 18
　air-filter/ionizer, 20
　capsules, 20
　Radiant Cream, 21
　Ride and Glide, 21
FSH. *See* follicle stimulating hormone

Gaia Herb Symposium, 4
gallbladder, 127–128, 224–225
gamma cells, 102. *See also* pancreas
Geller, Anderson, 9, 12
GH. *See* growth hormone
GHRH. *See* growth hormone releasing hormone
Gilday, Kate, 9
Gladstar, Rosemary, 5, 8, 41
glucagon, 101–102. *See also* pancreas
GnRH. *See* gonadotrophin releasing hormone
gonadotrophin releasing hormone (GnRH), 75. *See also* hypothalamus
Gotu Kola, 96
growth hormone (GH), 78–79. *See also* pituitary gland
growth hormone releasing hormone (GHRH), 75. *See also* hypothalamus

health signals. *See* organ/body correspondences
heart, 132–133, 230–231
herbal healing tools, 135–136
herbalism and activism, 14–15
herbalist, 11
　client files, 35
　composting, 15–16

using computer, 28–31
computer security and data protection, 31
consultation room and classroom, 36–39
desk area, 25–28
environmental consciousness and health, 14
financial considerations, 29–30
formula preparation area, 18–21
harmony with nature, 12–13
herbalism and activism, 14–15
herbarium box, 38
herb closet, 31–35
home-based practitioner, 16–17
laboratory, 39–41
library, 35–36
nutrition and self-care, 13–14
office space, 16–18, 21–25
organizing and nurturing herbal practice, 17–18
philosophy, 11–16
self-care for practitioners in healing arts, 15
sliding scale, 11
tincture preparation room, 39–41
work island, 18, 20
herbal practice, 17–18
herbarium box, 38
herb closet, 22, 31–35
herbs
　for adrenals, 85
　American Ginseng, 78, 85, 96
　Arnica flower, 77
　Burdock root, 77
　Chickweed, 85, 96
　Coleus, 96
　Gotu Kola, 96
　for hyperparathyroid, 92
　for hyperthyroid, 100
　for hypothalamus, 77–78
　for hypothyroid, 95–98
　Kelp, 95–96
　for kidneys, 131
　Licorice, 85, 97, 100
　Motherwort, 100

for ovaries, 109
for pancreas, 104–105
for parathyroid, 91
Passion Flower, 77, 97, 100
for pineal gland, 71–72
for pituitary, 80–81
Red Clover, 77
Rosemary, 97
for testes, 112
Vitex berry, 80, 97
home-based practitioner, 16–17
hormone, 66. *See also* endocrine cascade
HPA Axis, 73. *See also* hypothalamus
hydrocortisone, 82. *See also* adrenal glands
hyperparathyroidism, 92. *See also* endocrine cascade
hyperthyroidism, 98. *See also* endocrine cascade
  herbs for, 100
  indications for, 98–99
  nutrition for, 99–100
  supplements for, 100–101
hypothalamus, 72. *See also* endocrine cascade
  adrenocorticotropic hormone, 75
  bridging nervous and endocrine systems, 74
  corticotrophin releasing hormone, 75
  dopamine, 75
  follicle stimulating hormone, 75
  gonadotrophin releasing hormone, 75
  growth hormone releasing hormone, 75
  herbs for, 77–78
  hormones, 74–75
  HPA Axis, 73
  indications for, 76–77
  luteinizing hormone, 75
  nutritional support for, 77
  oxytocin, 74
  prolactin, 75
  somatostatin, 75
  supplements for, 78

  thyroid stimulating hormone, 75
  thytrophin releasing hormone, 74
hypothyroidism, 93. *See also* endocrine cascade
  herbs for, 95–98
  indications for, 93–94
  nutrition for, 94–95
  supplements for, 98

IBS. *See* irritable bowel syndrome
ICSH. *See* Interstitial cell stimulating hormone
insulin, 101. *See also* pancreas
intake form, 46–54. *See also* client intake
Interstitial cell stimulating hormone (ICSH), 110
invoice, 29, 30
irritable bowel syndrome (IBS), 76

Kapha, 44
Kelp, 95–96
kidneys, 131, 226–227

laboratory, 39–41
large intestine, 125–126, 220–221
  line examination, 189–191
lecithin, 101
LeSassier, William, 9
  tongue diagram, 166
LH. *See* luteinizing hormone
library, 35–36
Licorice, 85, 97, 100
life timeline, 45–46. *See also* client intake
Light, Phyllis D., 9
lip indications, 161–162
liver, 126–127, 222–223
lungs, 130–131, 228–229
luteinizing hormone (LH), 75, 107, 110. *See also* hypothalamus; ovaries

magnesium, 101
MAO inhibitors, 71
Matthew Wood tongue, 168
Matuza, Sarah, 9
McIntyre, Annie, 9

meditation
   for pineal gland, 69
   for thyroid, 87
melanocyte stimulating hormone (MSH), 79. *See also* pituitary gland
melatonin, 67, 68. *See also* pineal gland
men assessment, 61–63. *See also* client intake
moontime, 32
Motherwort, 100
mouth examination, 160–162
MSH. *See* melanocyte stimulating hormone

nature, harmony with, 12–13
noradrenalin. *See* norepinephrine
norepinephrine, 83. *See also* adrenal glands
nose examination, 157–158
nutrition and self-care, 13–14

office space
   choosing, 16–17
   using computer, 28–31
   creating, 21–25
   desk area, 23, 25–28
   entering professional space, 17–18
   herb closet, 22
   work island, 18, 20
oogenesis, 107. *See also* ovaries
organ/body correspondences, 123
   bladder, 131–132
   gallbladder, 127–128, 224–225
   heart, 132–133, 230–231
   kidneys, 131, 226–227
   large intestine, 125–126, 220–221
   liver, 126–127, 222–223
   lungs, 130–131, 228–229
   pelvic floor, 132, 232–233
   small intestine, 124–125, 218–219
   spleen/pancreas, 128–130, 216–217
   stomach, 123–124, 214–215
ovaries, 106. *See also* endocrine cascade
   esterone, 108
   estriol-DHEA, 107

   follicle simulating hormone, 107
   herbs for, 109
   indications for, 108–109
   luteinizing hormone, 107
   nutrition for, 109
   oogenesis, 107
   progesterone, 107
   supplements for, 110
oxytocin, 74. *See also* hypothalamus

pancreas, 101, 128–130. *See also* endocrine cascade
   alpha cells, 102
   amylin, 102
   beta cells, 102
   delta cells, 102
   gamma cells, 102
   glucagon, 101–102
   herbs for pancreas, 104–105
   indications for, 102–103
   insulin, 101
   nutrition for, 104
   pancreatic polypeptide, 102
   somatostatin, 102
   supplements for, 105–106
pancreatic polypeptide, 102. *See also* pancreas
parathyroid hormone (PTH), 90
parathyroidism, 90. *See also* endocrine cascade
   herbs for, 91
   indicators for, 90–91
   nutrition, 91
   supplements for, 91
Passion Flower, 77, 97, 100
pelvic floor, 132, 232–233
pericardium, 207
D-phenylalanine, 98
pineal gland, 66, 87. *See also* endocrine cascade
   amygdala, 68–69
   cycles of life, 66
   herbs for, 71–72
   indications for, 69–71
   meditation, 69
   melatonin, 67, 68

nutrition for, 71
pineal rings, 67
pineal to reproductive and basic emotional foundation, 67
serotonin, 68
supplements for, 72
pineal rings, 67
piton, 25
Pitta, 44
pituitary gland, 78. *See also* endocrine cascade
   follicle stimulating hormone, 79
   growth hormone, 78–79
   melanocyte stimulating hormone, 79
   supplements for, 80–81
   thyotrophin releasing hormone, 79
   thyroid stimulating hormone, 79
pituitary imbalance
   causes of, 79
   herbs for, 80–81
   indications for, 79–80
Polarity Therapy, 6
post traumatic stress disorder (PTSD), 76
PRL. *See* prolactin
progesterone, 107. *See also* ovaries
prolactin (PRL), 75. *See also* hypothalamus
PTH. *See* parathyroid hormone
PTSD. *See* post traumatic stress disorder
pupils, 152, 212

QuickBooks Pro Online, 28, 29

Radiant Cream, 21
Red Clover, 77
releasing factor (RF), 73
restorative and anabolic processes, 68
RF. *See* releasing factor
Ride and Glide, 21
Rosemary, 97

SAD. *See* seasonal affective disorder
Sanders, Karyn, 9
Schizandra, 78
scleral examination, 151
   client's view, 152
   conditions indicated by scleral color, 151–152
   below eyelid, 153–154
   pupils, 152
SCN. *See* suprachiasmatic nucleus
scybala, 196
seasonal affective disorder (SAD), 70
selenium, 98
   -rich foods, 95
self-care
   nutrition and, 13–14
   for practitioners in healing arts, 15
serotonin, 68. *See also* pineal gland
session, 43
   Ayurvedic medicine, 43
   doshas, 43
   Kapha, 44
   Pitta, 44
   Vata, 43–44
sliding scale, 11
small intestine, 124–125, 218–219
somatostatin, 75, 102. *See also* hypothalamus; pancreas
spleen, 128–130, 216–217
steroids
   androgenic, 82
stomach, 123–124, 214–215
stool analysis, 193
   color, 195
   consistency, 194–195
   ease of passage, 196–197
   factors in, 193
   and indications, 199–200
   odor, 196
   perfect bowel movement, 193, 194
   shape, 196
   stool color and indications, 200–201
   substances, 196
   transit time, 194
subacute thyroiditis, 99

Sumac tips, 80
suprachiasmatic nucleus (SCN), 68
Symposium, Gaia Herb, 4
symptoms and organ connections. *See* organ/body correspondences

testes, 110. *See also* endocrine cascade
    herbs for, 112
    indications, 111
    luteinizing hormone, 110
    nutrition for, 112
thiamine-rich foods, 77
Third Eye. *See* pineal gland
thyotrophin. *See* thyroid stimulating hormone
thyroid gland, 86. *See also* endocrine cascade
    environmental impacts for, 89–90
    general nutritional protection for, 87
    indications, 86
    meditation for, 87
    testing for, 87–89
    tongue indications, 181
thyroid stimulating hormone (TSH), 75, 79, 88. *See also* hypothalamus; pituitary gland
thyrotropin-releasing hormone (TRH), 74, 79. *See also* hypothalamus; pituitary gland
tincture preparation room, 39–41
tongue examination, 165
    areas of tongue and body, 166–167
    general analysis, 169–170
    indications associated with tongue coating, 178–179
    LeSassier tongue diagram, 166
    Matthew Wood tongue, 168
    specific indications, 171–177
    specific papillae indications, 179–180
    spirit of tongue, 169
    thyroid tongue indications, 181
    tongue body, 168
    tongue scraper, 165
tools of herbal healing, 135–136
tooth indications, 159–160
traditional medicine, 15
TRH. *See* thyrotropin-releasing hormone
triclosan, 89
Triple Heater, 207
tryptophan, 70
TSH. *See* thyroid stimulating hormone
tyrosine, 95
    L-tyrosine, 81

UBC. *See* Uterine Balancing Class
urine analysis, 203–204
Uterine Balancing Class (UBC), 54

Vata, 43–44
Vitamin B complex, 100
Vitamin C rich foods, 77
Vitamin D, 66
Vitex berry, 80, 97

Winston, David, 4, 8, 32
women assessment, 54–61. *See also* client intake
Women's Herbal Conference, 5
work island, 18, 20

www.ingramcontent.com/pod-product-compliance
Ingram Content Group UK Ltd.
Pitfield, Milton Keynes, MK11 3LW, UK
UKHW022359220226
468275UK00008BA/114